The Political Economy of Mental Illness in South Africa

The book describes key socio-political reforms that helped shape post-apartheid South Africa's mental health system.

The author interrogates how reforms shaped public, community-based services for people living with severe mental illness, and how features of this care has been determined, in part at least, by the relations between actors and structures in the state, private for-profit health care, and civil society spheres. A description of the development of South Africa's post-apartheid health system, and the contentions that emerge therein, sets the stage for an analysis of the country's most tragic human rights failure during its democratic period, namely the Life Esidimeni tragedy. The roots of the tragedy are not only framed as a loss of life and dignity as a result of political corruption and administrative mismanagement, but as a power differential that ultimately highlights an unjust system that relegates its most vulnerable citizens to commodities, without voice and without agency. The book concludes that the commodification of severe mental illness has been a product of neoliberal discourses that have shaped the economistic ways in which the post-apartheid South African state have governed poverty and severe mental illness.

This book will be of interest to scholars of health, social and economic policy in South Africa.

André J. van Rensburg is a senior researcher at the Centre for Rural Health, University of KwaZulu-Natal, South Africa, and a research fellow at the Centre for Health Systems Research & Development, University of the Free State, South Africa.

Routledge Studies in Health in Africa
Series Editor: Pieter Fourie

The Political Economy of Mental Illness in South Africa

André J. van Rensburg

Routledge
Taylor & Francis Group
LONDON AND NEW YORK

First published 2021
by Routledge
2 Park Square, Milton Park, Abingdon, Oxon OX14 4RN

and by Routledge
52 Vanderbilt Avenue, New York, NY 10017

Routledge is an imprint of the Taylor & Francis Group, an informa business

British Library Cataloguing-in-Publication Data
A catalogue record for this book is available from the British Library

Library of Congress Cataloging-in-Publication Data
A catalog record has been requested for this book

ISBN: 978-0-367-19263-1 (hbk)
ISBN: 978-0-367-68329-0 (pbk)
ISBN: 978-0-429-20145-5 (ebk)

Typeset in Times New Roman
by Newgen Publishing UK

For Lize

Contents

Prologue

The core ideas in this book are rooted in a doctoral dissertation, completed at Stellenbosch University and Ghent University, in 2018. The timing of my doctoral research fell in almost perfect sequence with the Life Esidimeni tragedy, and, while my topic focused on mental health care in South Africa, the events could not be adequately translated into the research and dissertation. This book offered an opportunity to reflect on the Life Esidimeni events more fully, in an attempt to move beyond linear explanations of individual incompetence, greed or cruelty. Much is left to explore, and this is a very small start to a longer trajectory in studying the South African mental health system. Arthur Kleinman's (1998, 358):

> So daunting is my subject, so limited my skills, that I must beg your indulgence with my overreaching. I do so not to amuse you with a display of my pretensions, but because of a keen sense that there is in this subject so much that matters for all of us.

Chapters 1, 2, 4, 6, and 7 contain revised sections from the following published papers:

Janse van Rensburg, A., Wouters, E., Fourie, P., van Rensburg, D. and Bracke, P., 2018. Collaborative mental health care in the bureaucratic field of post-apartheid South Africa. Health Sociology Review, 27(3), pp. 279–293.

Janse van Rensburg, A., Khan, R., Fourie, P. and Bracke, P., 2019. Politics of mental health care in post-apartheid South Africa. Politikon, 46(2), pp. 192–205.

Chapter 3 has previously been published as the following:

Janse van Rensburg, A., Petersen, I., Wouters, E., Engelbrecht, M., Kigozi, G., Fourie, P., van Rensburg, D. and Bracke, P., 2018. State and non-state mental health service collaboration in a South African district: a mixed methods study. Health Policy and Planning, 33(4), pp. 516–527.

Chapter 5 has previously been published as the following:

Janse van Rensburg, A., Khan, R., Wouters, E., van Rensburg, D., Fourie, P. and Bracke, P., 2018. At the coalface of collaborative mental health care: A qualitative study of governance and power in district-level service provision in South Africa. The International Journal of Health Planning and Management, 33(4), pp. 1121–1135.

These publications also appear in the following dissertation:

Janse van Rensburg, A. 2018. Governance and Power in Mental Health Integration Processes in South Africa. Doctoral Dissertation. Stellenbosch University and Ghent University. Supervisors: Prof Pieter Fourie and Prof Dr. Piet Bracke.

Acknowledgment

This work was supported by the Wellcome Trust [219675/Z/19/Z]; National Institute For Health Research [GHRU 16/136/54]; and National Institute for Mental Health [1U19MH113191-01]. The views expressed in this publication are those of the author and not necessarily those of the funders.

1 Introduction

On 19 October 2017, Reverend Joseph Maboe, in the most public of spaces, told the world what happened with his son Hendrick Ramtodi Maboe, known as "Billy". Billy was one of a group of people with severe mental and neurological conditions that have come to be known as the Life Esidimeni victims. Following a highly controversial chain of decisions by the Gauteng Department of Health in 2015–2016, a large group of patients were removed from the private, subsidised facilities of Life Health care and moved into the care of a number of organisations purportedly specialising in care for severe and debilitating conditions. After a number of investigations, it was found that 144 people died due to neglect – some remain missing to this day. The absolute horror, the systemic contexts within which the Life Esidimeni events were rendered possible, were laid bare in thousands of pieces of commentary and, most pressingly, in the narratives of the victims' families. In a key extract from Reverend Maboe's testimony at the Life Esidimeni public arbitration hearings in 2017, we see a searing indictment of South Africa's post-apartheid mental health system:

Box 1.1

Billy looked hungry. Billy looked dehydrated. He was dry. He could hardly speak ... Billy was a jolly person. He could speak, when at Life Esidimeni, when they bring him from the wards to come and see me, when I visited him at Life Esidimeni, we were always accommodated in a hall, families. He will just laugh and hug me and when he just enter there he will say "Papa, you have come, thank you very much that you have come!", and but on that particular day, on the 16th of July, Billy was as dumb, and found like I don't know. He could hardly say a word, and so...he had to hug me, and then he was shivering there. I could see that he was going to fall and then we supported him, and they said "Bring him a chair", and they brought him this green chair that he's sitting on, and also a plastic, a refuge plastic bag to sit on.

And they, he was there and said whilst we're still talking there, he said I'm thirsty, I want water and the old nurse said "No, no, no we're not giving you water, because he's wetting himself." He's peeing his trousers and so on. I could believe that, because how he was stinking with dirt. No, they didn't bring him anything. He was not given anything to drink…he's wetting himself and that's the end of the story. So, we said no, let's go and sit out in the sun and then we went out and took his chair along and then we supported him, put him on this chair outside. It was a bit warmish outside, and he asked me "Did you bring me some food Papa? Some chips?", because he liked chips. He liked bread and Coke. I said "No, we haven't brought those things, because we are coming to fetch you, because we brought you new clothes." Tekkies, a lumber jacket and jerseys and so on, and then we sat outside there and he said I want something to eat. So, I saw somebody there and called him. Now the crux of the matter was that while we were sitting outside, waiting for the man who was going to buy chips and whatever, the process of starting to renovate was starting on that particular, I don't know whether it started on that particular day or it had already started some days back, because they were putting on security fence. They building walls around and these poor fellows, we could not see them properly because they were that side, but this side because we could see them, some of them were on that side at the entrance of the car. Some of them were basking in the sun there … The other patients were just – you know what mental patients are. They will ask you can you give us two rand to go and buy a cigarette. I want something to go and buy, they were just screaming at us you see. One of them was singing there, he was just singing an endless anthem which I cannot remember, but he was singing for the whole time sitting there around us and … They were confined in that particular area. This was the house here and on the side here, on the side of the house, at the end of the house, they put up a fence or a brick wall and now the brick wall was being built up on the side here so that they cannot jump onto the other property.

I sent somebody who took a very long time, more than half an hour or quarter of an hour, because you know Hammanskraal, they are depending on tuck shops which I don't know what types of tuckshops are, and then he came back after a while, when we were already worried that that fellow is gone with our money. So, fortunately he came back. He came back with a packet of chips and a bottle of Coke. The chips were dry. They were old, and so the poor fellow because he was so hungry he just took that plastic and started to, he wanted to eat even the plastic, the way he was hungry, and we said to, I said to my cousin, he said to me I want to go to the loo. So, they asked him to go right around the house so they open up the gate, so he went right around the house and then he came back. I said I also want to go to the loo, but he said "Ramagolo, please. I'm begging you, don't go to the back. Don't go to the back of this house. It's horrible." What is happening? He said the garage, these people there are in the big garage. There are beds, 40 beds were lined up. There was no privacy. There was no washing basin. There was nothing. It was only those beds, and a few blankets I think. I don't want to go and see the mess behind there, but what you could see, there's a pit toilet right at the corner there … and we said to ourselves how can these poor patients use a pit toilet. It's really not safe for them, and we continued with my niece to ask ourselves a lot of questions which we could not get answers.

Then we told the old lady that, the old nurse that we are coming to fetch Billy, because we see that he is not well. We are going to take him home. But she insisted that you cannot take Billy away, because the doctor must see him. He must sign some documents and also the social worker must come, sign some documents … you are not allowed to take him. I said now really, but really, we feel that we must take him away, but she insisted that no you can't. So, I said okay, we'll respect you and your profession and your authority. We'll respect that, we won't take Billy away, but we left that place at about something, round about twelve or so, but one thing that hurt us at that time, there was no sign of lunch, because normally at Esidimeni when you go there, Life Esidimeni Randfontein, when you go there round about that time, twelve, they are already on lunch. But you could see that these poor people, these poor patients, did not even have breakfast in the first place. Now it's already that time, eleven o'clock or so to twelve. There was no sign of lunch. There was nothing. Nothing. So probably Billy was lucky to have that packet of chips and drink.

So, we said now we are going to go. So we left all the clothes that we had for him and we said okay, we are leaving now and we'll probably come back on Monday or we'll hear from you, staff nurse from you, and you will tell us the position, but she said "We are going to take Billy to the clinic on Monday, and we'll give you the feedback when we come back from the clinic." Then I ask her how do you take them to the clinic. She said "No, we are using a bakkie, and then those who are sick as Billy is, he will be sitting in front and the rest, the others will be sitting at the back." Okay, no thank you very much. So, we left that place with very heavy hearts when we saw that, but I said to my niece, I said to him "I don't see Billy living more days than what he see him here", and we left that place with heavy hearts. Saying if Billy is like this, we didn't see the other fellows who probably were like him, but the others that we saw roaming around in the yard, they were there, they were sort of just as you know the mental patients. They are restless, they are not at one place. Some of them were just basking in the sun there. And then on Monday Tuesday, we got a phone call. From Bopelong NGO. They said Billy has been admitted at Jubilee Hospital. You need to make it a point to come and see him. His condition is not really so good.

The time we left Randfontein, it was the time when Billy died and I prepared to, I had taken holy communion along with me. I had holy oil to go an anoint him. But when I was told that he is no more, I just said ja.

> I had no other words, and then I said "Okay Sister, thank you very much for your information. We'll go back home and then go and arrange, because tomorrow it's Saturday." There is nothing that we can do. We won't be able to come and collect the body, because the mortuaries are closed, the undertakers are busy and we asked that we can we get his clothing, his pajamas whatever he went with to the hospital and she said "No okay, do you want to see him?" We said yes, definitely we want to see him. I thought she was saying that Billy is already in the mortuary. But most unfortunately, or luckily, he was still screened in the ward. So, she took us around into the ward and then she unscreened the bed and then I saw Billy was no more, and I started praying because I could not anoint him, I could not give him holy communion. I prayed for … his soul and offered him to God and then went home. His grandparents, ancestors, everybody, said "accept Billy." Lord, accept Billy's soul. May his soul rest in peace and then I said to Billy we are coming to fetch you my son. We'll be coming on Monday and I gave blessing, and we left. We said no, we want to have his belongings. They open up the drawer there. We took out his clothes, his shoes and everything. Then we went back to Bophelong, which I didn't call Bophelong. I call it death … ["Bophelong" means life].

In this gut-wrenching, incredibly rich piece of narrative, multiple themes emerge of profound disfunction. Billy's corporeal breakdown is vividly illustrated by his speech regression, his extreme hunger and general demeanour. His hunger was especially vivid, reaching a peak when devouring an old packet of chips. The sheer inhumanity of his care can be seen in the coldness of the nurse denying him water due to his incontinence, and making him sit on a refuse bag. The Reverend's observation of the "security upgrades" at the facility, the erecting of fencing to keep the patients inside, speaks to the well-known discourse of containment that has haunted psychiatry since its very beginning. The pit toilet reminds one of a key post-apartheid indicator of social justice and progress, a frequent flash point in public protests and a persistent challenge to state legitimacy. The stacking of 40 beds in the garage – a space reserved for the keeping of possessions and equipment – with no sign of personal belongings recalls memories of concentration camp settings, where all individuality and subjectivity is stripped from its inhabitants. The refusal from the nurse to let Billy go underlines his status as a possession, rather than an individual with inherent freedom. His release was further attached to the bureaucracies of medical gatekeeping, the power of which is so woven into our daily lives that we just accept it as an unmoveable boundary. Billy died alone in a district hospital on the outskirts of Tswane, denied participation in the community of cultural and spiritual practices that is such a key dimension of death in South Africa. His father's resignation at his death, and changing of the interpretation of the Bophelong community organisation's meaning, highlights an inevitability in South Africa's mental health system, and also plays on the irony of Life Esidimeni's translation from isiZulu, namely "place of dignity". The movement between spaces of dignity and disgrace is a fundamental feature of South Africa's post-apartheid reality, and key to getting to grips of why the system fails the vulnerable so completely.

This book is a starting step towards better understanding the complex dynamics inherent in providing mental health care to people living with debilitating, severe mental and neurological conditions. During its post-apartheid period, South Africa's scholarly community have produced an immense body of knowledge, its advocates have continued to lobby for the rights of people living with mental illness, and the government has made important legislative and policy gains in improving public mental health. South Africa has been an active participant in global health governance shifts, particularly in its engagement with the World Health Organization (WHO) and the Movement for Global Mental Health. Despite the many gains made, the Life Esidimeni events rocked the mental health community and set in motion an important period of self-reflection – no doubt made more prescient by unfolding towards the back end of South Africa's first comprehensive mental health policy, one that took decades of research and lobbying to formulate and put in place, with the same lofty promises brought by South Africa's democratic transition. It exposed an important blind spot in our current focus in looking at mental health systems, namely the increasing salience of political economy in shaping the structure and outcomes of care. The mental health care narrative thus far has been driven by psychiatry and psychology, and the absence of a more interdisciplinary perspective from disciplines such as anthropology, sociology and political science is telling. Far from being comprehensive, or empirical, this book is an exploration in how a wide body of critical scholarship can help us understand the deep and persistent dynamics that puts a boot on the neck of people with severe mental and neurological conditions. Rather than adopting an analysis rooted in scientism, we apply key concepts from a range of critical perspectives to developments in mental health care during South Africa's post-apartheid period.

What is meant by "severe mental and neurological conditions"

The mere mention of mental illness and all its variants opens up a plethora of political, biomedical and philosophical problems. More than perhaps any other set of human afflictions, mental illness has, under the names of "madness", "insanity", "lunacy", and "mental illness", historically provoked a wide variety of often contradictory reactions (Eghigian 2010). After all, "psychiatric concepts are products of social forces" (Moncrieff 2014, 591). Terms such as "mental illness", "mental disability", "mental conditions", "mental distress" etc. are often used interchangeably. And while we are more successful, relatively speaking, in treating symptoms of some disorders with medication and other therapies, the complex roots of mental illness remain elusive (Coleborne & Smith 2020). As described by Bruce Scott (Scott 2016, np):

> When one uses the term "mental health", in a context where it means everything (e.g., concerning mental distress) the concept of health and ill-health subsumes the all of the context. However, the concept has so much slippage when subjected to a detailed critical analysis, it deteriorates into a phantasm that continually haunts in the background, because the concept cannot contain or represent in an ideal way, when it reduces or reifies human experience in such a way.

Defining mental illness is rooted in an enduring legacy of controversy, and writing a book involving mental illness as a focus means engaging with this controversy. It is important to position the concept of mental illness within the boundaries of professional power within which it has been cast in the modern era. Accordingly, "psychiatry does not just understand and treat, it also defines and delimits. That is to say, psychiatric categories and practices of diagnosis help set the boundaries (and often blur the boundaries) of who is or is not a suitable case for (what kind of) treatment" (Rose 2019, p. 6). Beyond the power of mental health professionals, mental illness – especially in its more severe guises – is often determined by structures beyond the formal health system, for instance by police officers (Boyd & Kerr 2016). The global mainstay for expounding the meaning and diagnosis of mental illness (and related terms) is the Diagnostic and Statistical Manual of Mental Disorders (DSM), now in its fifth edition (American Psychiatric Association 2013). Ever since its first publication in 1952, the DSM has had substantial influence in global discourses on psychiatric nosology and treatment. However, the "Bible" of psychiatry has had pushback following each of its versions, and its most recent iteration – the DSM-5, published in 2013, have perhaps had more intense resistance. The result of decades of synthesis and effort, the fifth edition was produced after five years of work by a team of 397 participants in 13 working groups, 6 study groups, and a specialist task team led by the American Psychological Association, the National Institutes of Health, the National Institute of Drug Abuse, the National Institute of Alcoholism and Alcohol Abuse, the World Health Organization (WHO), and the World Psychiatric Association (Vahia 2013). Despite this impressive effort, the DSM has been the subject of regular critique. The main criticisms were rooted in the use of phenotypic categories with little biological basis, conflating psychiatric pathology with human conditions deemed contextually appropriate, creating categories when dimensional line could be more accurate, and not shifting the boundaries between some disorders (e.g. bipolar and major depressive disorders; Gitlin & Miklowitz 2014). It has been noted that it is very much skewed towards Western psychiatry, with high levels of disparities between its content and approach, and individual psychiatric practice (Pickersgill 2012).

Concerns were also raised over the "medicalisation" of normality in line with pharmaceutical intervention (Pickersgill 2013). Significantly, the National Institutes for Mental Health (NIMH) abandoned using the DSM in favour of developing their own version, the Research Domain Criteria (RDoC) approach. The other major diagnostic system – the *International Classification of Diseases*, 11th Revision (ICD-11) – is however limited in similar ways. A central difficulty in pinning down a rigorous definition of mental illness – especially in comparison to other medical ailments with more clear-cut biological roots – is complicated by differing stances in empirically derived evidence for biological and physiological aetiology of mental disorders in psychiatric discourse. While some claim that there are little to no biological evidence for mental disorders (Burstow 2015; Rose 2013), such claims have more recently been challenged by a growing body of evidence of possible genetic influences on mental disorders, for instance genetic overlap between attention-deficit/hyperactivity disorder and bipolar disorder (van Hulzen et al., 2017) and the effects of a structural brain abnormality, caused by a genetic mutation during adolescence, on the formation of schizophrenia (Luo et al., 2019). This is part of broader shifts towards embracing brain-based, biomedical approaches to classifying mental illness (Rose, 2019). Indeed, an editorial in The Lancet promotes this idea further:

> The furor surrounding new versions of the two major classification systems in psychiatry (DSM-5 and ICD-11) is giving way to a more fundamental debate about the nature and origin of mental illness. While recognising the pragmatic benefits of symptom-based approaches, clinicians and researchers look forward to a new era of diagnosis and treatment based on underlying cause. … The future of psychiatry looks set to change from the current model, in which ADHD, bipolar disorder, or schizophrenia are considered as totally different illnesses, to a model in which the underlying cause of a spectrum of symptoms determines the treatment.
>
> (The Lancet 2013, p. 1878)

Groopman's (2019) suggestion that "when pathogenesis is absent, historical events and cultural shifts have an outsized influence on prevailing views on causes and treatments" rings true. Fundamentally, as Ian Hacking (2013) pointed out, our attempts to classify mental illness are inherently flawed due to our conceptualisations (especially the DSM) being based on a botanical model, rather than adequately reflecting the true nature and realities of the varieties of mental illnesses. In short, mental illness cannot be neatly stacked into clear-cut boxes. Diagnosis and definition are made all the more difficult given that there are no known biological markers with which to pin down mental conditions (Rose 2013). While this certainly challenges analyses of mental illness, Susan Sontag (1978, 58) highlights the importance of engaging in this project as a political struggle:

> The notion that a disease can be explained only by a variety of causes is precisely characteristic of thinking about diseases whose causation is not [italicised in the original text] understood. And it is diseases thought to be multi-determined (that is, mysterious) that have the widest possibilities as metaphors for what is felt to be socially or morally wrong.

Without wading into the murky waters of pinning down mental illness as a concept, and for the sake of pragmatism, we accept that the definition of mental illness is closely intertwined with policy, with the most important consideration being the severity of impairment (Goldman & Grob 2006). The National Mental Health Policy Framework and Strategic Plan 2013–2020 defines mental illness as "a positive diagnosis of a mental health related illness in terms of diagnostic criteria made by a mental health care practitioner authorized to make such diagnosis" (South African National Department of Health 2013, 7), which strongly and overtly highlights professional power and diagnosis. Ultimately, "we are limited by our ignorance on two major issues: (1) the biological underpinnings and proper boundaries of psychiatric disorders; and (2) how to set the proper balance between being inclusive enough to ensure the proper treatment of suffering individuals while not overpathologizing human conditions…all diagnostic systems including DSM-5 and ICD-11 will be inherently imperfect creations with compromises based on our field's ignorance, not necessarily wilful thoughtlessness" (Gitlin & Miklowitz 2014, 90). A neatly formulated definition of mental illness lies far beyond the scope and purpose of this book. Rather, we acknowledge the complexities, pluralities, conflicting and converging interests attached to the term (and its related iterations). For pragmatic reasons, this book focuses on mental illness in terms of "official" responses to it as a social phenomenon, the ways in which states exercise power over individuals in particular ways, particularly through policy and legislation. No claims are made regarding the "truth" of mental illness. I carefully acknowledge that there is a degree of validity in psychiatric diagnosis in selected conditions, but also that there is a fair amount of evidence of psychiatric hegemony, critiques that highlight a troubling relationship between diagnostic power and professional, pharmacological and capitalist interests. An enduring deficiency in responses to mental illness is a lack of engagement with subjective experience and cultural manifestations of disease, particularly in the era of Global Mental Health. Accordingly, terms like "mental disorder", "mental illness", "psychiatric disorder", "mental condition" and associated terminologies are understood interchangeably, a specific perception of mental vulnerability by the South African state, professional societies, news media and broader public in discourses leading up to and following the Life Esidimeni tragedy. In general, we refer to people with severe mental and neurological conditions, explicitly not referring to complete diagnostic criteria, but rather to a domain of illnesses that substantially inhibit an individual from participating in social, economic and political life, thought to be rooted in the brain, neurological system or mental sphere. This uses "people" to denote individual experience as well as communal, shared experience; qualifies "suffering" in terms of individual experience of psychological and, often, physiological, misery; "mental and neurological conditions" to allow for the inclusion of afflictions deemed to be mental in nature (e.g. psychosis, depression, anxiety) as well as neurological conditions stemming from the brain, spine and the nerves (epilepsy, Parkinson's disease and stroke); and – perhaps the most important part of this characterization – the term "severe". It is precisely here where states intervene, where public responses such as stigma, violence and exploitation converge. Severity in this sense means that someone is considered to be unable to do "routine" or "normal" everyday activities, including more basic activities such as cooking, cleaning and self-care, as well as more advanced activities such as participating in the labour market. An important focus here is on the perceived inherent *ability* of sufferers from mental illness to participate in everyday life, an assumption that have increasingly been contested by disability scholars (disability studies has arguably progressed much more than mental health sciences in promoting a critical discourse of the meaning of illness and impairment). Severity is something that is determined – usually by a mental health professional – and the principal consideration of the degree of assistance a person needs. It is a central determining factor in deciding where the person receives care – in their home, at a caretaker's home, a non-governmental facility, or a government institution. It is precisely here – the management of severity – where the Life Esidimeni events unfolded, and where the heart of this book is aimed. Accordingly, we reflect on pertinent dimensions of the political economy of *severe* mental and neurological disorders in South Africa, a population of people very much exposed to misfires in the health system machinery. The focus is therefore not on what is termed "common mental disorders", conditions with a lower degree of severity, though this grouping is the subject of a whole other political economy under neoliberal conditions.[1] We therefore dispense with the mind-body dualism that has allowed sociologists and other social scientists to focus on mental illness as either a brain or body problem, towards accepting that a fair degree of subjectivity is wrapped up in these complexities. In short, "viewed from the decidedly ordinary practices of everyday experience, human conditions certainly have a biology, but they have a history, a politics, an economics, and they reflect cultural and subjective differences" (Kleinman 1998, 371).

Making sense of mental health care in contemporary times

Applying the idea that "contexts matter", and that an interdisciplinary approach based on a critical worldview and a pragmatic method can offer much to our understanding of the ways in which we as a post-apartheid society have responded to severe mental and neurological conditions. This inevitably requires a degree of selectiveness, and the issues raised in the following chapters are not meant to be comprehensive. Rather, it is a subjective reflection on key dimensions in mental health care scholarship that have been neglected in the South African case. By highlighting specific areas of investigation, the book aims to open a body of exploration of South Africa's mental health system dynamics, rooted in sociology, political science, critical theory, and social anthropology, to complement the bulk of current scholarship tethered to the fields of psychiatry, psychology and epidemiology.

Importantly, we take a step back and attempt to describe South Africa's mental health system in more generous terms, by not focusing on state-provided services, but also the critical, but underappreciated, non-state spheres of service division. In terms of public mental health, this means services aimed at the strata of the population who do not have the socio-economic means to access the for-profit private sphere, and whose interests are often carried by civil society. South Africa has a pluralistic health system, meaning that multiple sectors are involved in service provision, led by the state. However, we need to define and delineate what is meant by "state" and "non-state". As discussed below, non-state service providers can further be distinguished in terms of for-profit and non-profit motives. As will become apparent later in the article, the lines drawn between these service providers often become blurry, and the following descriptions are meant to – in broad strokes – anchor the discussion in particular groups of actors.

The state is the steward of health care in South Africa, with the official responsibility for strategic leadership in mental health care provision (Coovadia, Jewkes, Barron, Sanders, & McIntyre 2009b). State-managed health facilities provide health care to the (uninsured) bulk of the South African population. This responsibility is legally underwritten in section 27 of the Constitution of the Republic of South Africa (South African Government 1996), as well as in the National Health Act (South African Government 2004). The concept of "the state" and state institutions therefore emerge as a central unit of analysis. Weber (Weber 1947) conceived of the state as a political organisation with compulsory association, within a given territory whose administrative staff successfully maintains a monopoly of legitimate use of physical force that is essential to the enforcement of its order. Following this definition, Mann (Mann 1993) surmised that the state (1) is territorially centralised; (2) contains two dualities: place and persons, and centre and territory; (3) institutions are differentiated in order to undertake different functions for different interest groups; and (4) engages in geopolitics with other states, due to its delimited territorial nature. The state has further been described as "a relatively unified ensemble of socially embedded, socially regularized, and strategically selective institutions and organizations", which operates in a given territorial area (Jessop 2016, 49). Without wading into the depth and breadth of conceptions of the state – it certainly comprises "whole libraries of historical investigation, and whole bookshops of radical critique" (Rabinow & Rose 2003, 5) – we will indicate a break with more traditional views of the state. Governmentality scholars have critiqued the Weberian notion of the state, arguing that "the state possessed neither the unity nor the functionality ascribed to it; it was a mythical abstraction which has assumed a particular place in the field of government" (Rose & Miller 2010a, 175). Analyses of the modern state focused on its inevitable tendency to centralise, control, regulate and manage, an approach rooted in 19th century social theory "which accords 'the state' a quite illusory necessity, functionality and territorialisation" (Rose 1999, 18). Taking these considerations into account, the present examination approaches the state in a Bourdieusian fashion, namely that it is not a coordinated and monolithic ensemble, but rather a "splintered space of forces vying over the definition and distribution of public goods" (Wacquant 2010, 200). In Bourdieu's language, we approach the state as a field, more specifically, a bureaucratic field, where the state is a "culmination of a process of concentration of different species of capital" and the power dynamics that it elicits (Bourdieu 1994, 5). Within the bureaucratic field, traditionally non-state institutions operate, and in the South African mental health care context these are private for-profit care and private not-for-profit care.

Private for-profit care can be termed "non-state" in that it does not operate under the direct auspices of the state government, although service providers still operate under the legislative sovereignty of the state. Driven by profit and market forces, these include hospital groups, individual, and group medical practices. Post-apartheid developments saw a significant increase in non-insured use of private medical care (Development Bank of Southern Africa 2008; Harrison 2009b). This increase has especially been due to a growing realisation of the effects of the HIV/AIDS epidemic on the workforce, corporate social investment, and an increase in employed, uninsured people (Wolvaardt, van Niftrik, Beira, Mapham, & Tienie 2008). These factors, along with a favourable policy environment, led to a rapid expansion of private health providers, especially hospital groups (H. Van Rensburg 2012).

Private not-for-profit care: As in many low-to-middle income countries (LMICs), the civil society sector in South Africa has been invaluable in providing health care to those not able to access certain services, especially private-for-profit services. Here the terms NGO and CSO are used interchangeably, as umbrella terms, one which encapsulates a range of different organisations across the social, political and economic spectrum, including faith-based, community-based, welfare or charity, and development organisations (International Labour Organization 2013) – essentially organisations not subsumed under traditional state institutions, with the primary logic of community service over profit-making. Traditional healers – especially prolific in providing mental health care in some areas of South Africa – are also considered as CSOs (Wolvaardt et al. 2008). CSOs have been especially instrumental in the provision of residential/institutionalisation services for people living with mental illness (WHO 2008b). In the relative absence of psychiatrists, psychologists and mental health nurses generally and particularly in the public sector, CSOs such as professional organisations, religious groups, patient support groups, and traditional healers have significantly contributed to mental, emotional, and spiritual well-being in poor communities (Wolvaardt et al. 2008). CSOs further act as liaison between families and government agencies for grant access, by providing material support to families waiting for grant application processing and catalysing government action in expediting application processes (Rosenberg, Hartwig, & Merson 2008).

Looking at the relationships between these three dimensions – the state, the private for-profit sector, and civil society – not only pragmatic issues relating to service provision, collaboration and outcomes of care emerge, but also more fundamental questions related to justice, freedom and democracy. This is telling in the Life Esidimeni tragedy, where all three sectors were thrown into the public sphere, that helped lift the veil on some more subtle variations of power.

In this sense, an increasingly important consideration in the ways in which these relations are shaped by neoliberalism, specifically how it has played out in South Africa. In this vein, the neoliberal project has very much been transnational, exhibiting three broad dimensions (Satgar 2012):

1. A capital growth model favouring financialization and marketisation through various liberal policy mechanisms
2. The fostering of a global market civilisation built on individualism and competition
3. A form of governance – referred to as governmentality – a "conduct of conduct", a way in which citizens are made into self-governing subjects

These dimensions are built on the assumption that "the contemporary state form is remade by transnational neoliberalism not to serve the political subjectivity of citizens but to ensure that the sovereignty of capital is protected from risk" (Satgar 2012, 40).

Neoliberalism's renewed attention after the 2008 global economic crisis has yet again been revived in the wake of the global COVID-19 pandemic, both events which forced reflections on justice, freedom and democracy. It has highlighted well-known warnings of the incompatibility of neoliberal values and those of liberal democracy, including notions of power sharing, political participation, and individual liberties (Brown 2003). Importantly in the South African context, the neoliberal project instigated "decollectivisation", a reconfiguration of the social in the image of the entrepreneurial individual, that ultimately meant that collective and shared notions of suffering were reduced to individual victimhood, undermining the principles of social justice following the Truth and Reconciliation Commission (Bowsher 2020). Neoliberal influencing did not only have economic consequences but also significantly shaped the mental health system and induced a justice that is retributive and restorative, but not distributive, thereby perpetuating poor systems of care. In this way, neoliberal discourses have gutted both democratic principles and democratic morality, particularly by framing scandals such as Life Esidimeni as a result of political miscalculation rather than in terms of institutional morality (Brown 2003; Fassin 2015).

Structure of the book

Author Adam Hochschild noted once in a lecture that all books – fiction and nonfiction – should follow the same simple recipe in order to reach a broader public. Ever since Homer, the basic ingredients of Characters, Scenes and Plot have been an enduringly effective way to convey a message (Hochschild 2014). Accordingly, we introduce characters in a structural sense – the state, for-profit private care, and civil society. As will become apparent, the obvious missing character in this narrative is that of people with severe mental and neurological conditions, and the glaring gap in this field of scholarship remains. The scenes are apparent: An overview of post-apartheid South African mental health care (Chapter 2); an empirical description of its contemporary structure (Chapter 3); a discussion on the relations between the state and civil society in the mental health system (Chapter 4); an empirical exploration of the dimensions of power that emerge within these relations (Chapter 5); an example of the consequences of major mental health system failure, drawing from the Life Esidimeni case (Chapter 6); a discussion of the implications of neoliberalism on South Africa's mental health system (Chapter 7); and finally, a reflection on what this narrative means for the future, and how we might want to start thinking about mental health system reform (Chapter 8). Following a classic literary plot structure, Chapters 1–5 provides a kind of exposition, setting the stage for the main points under discussion, ending with rising action in discussing the NAWONGO and SASSA court cases. Chapter 6, with the Life Esidimeni case at the centre, unquestionably plays the part of climax, where the true intentions of the characters and the consequences for people with severe mental and neurological conditions are unveiled. Falling action is then unpacked under the guise of Chapter 7, where the theoretical tenets of care under neoliberalism is explored. Finally, we reach a degree of resolution and denouement in Chapter 8, where we reflect on the narrative presented, and mull over possible themes that require further exploration.

In this way, we are attempting here to illustrate a narrative of mental health care, specifically focusing on the politics involved when we as a society develop and foster systems of care for those with conditions on the more severe end of the spectrum. Ultimately this book is a subjective attempt to make sense of the structural reasons that lie behind events such as the Life Esidimeni case, specifically in terms of our collective response as a society to the most vulnerable. It is rather a very limited overview of South Africa's post-apartheid trajectory in reforming its mental health system, focusing on the positioning of and tensions between state and non-state role players. This positioning and tension in mental health service delivery is exemplified by key formal and informal tensions. This focus on the political economy of severe mental illness in South Africa is an attempt to provide a complimentary perspective on challenges in mental health service provision, beyond the usual narrative that points to a lack of mental health specialists as the main culprit. As will become clear, it is impossible to disentangle the ways in which people with severe mental illness are "managed" from key social structures and processes. By interrogating South Africa's post-apartheid policy landscape, its health and social care systems, and particular discourses of care and responsibility, we can begin to understand the enduring roots of care that remains uncoordinated, inefficient and of poor quality – the level of care that results in physical and mental degradation, indignity, and death.

Note

1 The contested nature of depression and its treatment persists, especially with the advent of Global Mental Health and more emphasis of depression in the Global Burden of Disease Study. It is a central component of mental health screening tools and diagnostic manuals, and the efficacy of antidepressants have been the subject of quite literally thousands of clinical trials. The results of these trials have been routinely assessed in meta analyses, which tend to show consistent – if low to modest – effect size differences between different antidepressants and placebos. However, unlike in the case of other drugs whose trials led to a degree of consensus on their efficacy, antidepressants have been the subject of intense debate. Two of the more prominent critics are Joanna Moncrieff (a psychiatrist) and Irving Kirsch (a psychologist). They claim that selective serotonin reuptake inhibitors have an advantage over placebos, stating that statistical significance is not the same as clinical significance. They also attribute the effects that do arise from these trials to aspects of trial methodology (Joanna Moncrieff & Kirsch 2005; J. Moncrieff, Wessely, & Hardy 2004). In their view, there is no proof that antidepressants have any action on mood neurobiology (J. Moncrieff 2008). Irving Kitsch, after analysing data from the Federal Drug Administration agency, came to the conclusion that trials testing the efficacy of antidepressants were biased and tended to hide unfavourable results, perpetuating the idea that depression is caused by a chemical brain imbalance and that antidepressants are effective treatments for depression (Kirsch 2011). Differences between the efficacy of antidepressants and placebos that do increase in trials are due to a function of baseline severity; the response of extremely depressed people participating in trials is the result of decreased responsiveness to the placebo rather than an increase in responsiveness to the medication (Kirsch et al. 2008). Kirsch's analyses have been challenged for suffering from key flaws, selecting reporting and unjustified conclusions (Fountoulakis & Möller 2011). The debate continues, with recent meta analyses again claiming that antidepressants do not sufficiently outweigh placebos in terms of efficiency, that alternative treatments such as psychotherapy produce the same benefits with lower relapse rates without drug side effects (Kirsch 2019) and that the small benefits of selective serotonin reuptake inhibitors are outweighed by an increase the risk of adverse events (Jakobsen et al. 2017). While the robustness of trial methods has been improved in recent times, antidepressants still tend to have a modest 10% advantage over placebos (an effect size of 0.30), and newer generation drugs have little to no advantage over older antidepressants (Khan & Brown 2015; Khan, Fahl Mar, Faucett, Khan Schilling, & Brown 2017).

The central contention between the two camps is not necessarily disagreement on the validity of trials or robustness in measurement, but rather about the nature of depression itself. Moncrieff is highly critical of the claim that depression is a biological disease, the result of a chemical imbalance in the brain. This narrative was manufactured to exert more control over populations and to serve the interests of neoliberal agendas of global pharmaceutical companies. "The misconception that mental illness can be cured by drugs discourages the provision of decent services that recognise and respect difference and disability and promotes instead the notion that people can be drugged into some sort of conformity or passivity" (J. Moncrieff 2008, 220). Nikolas Rose (2003, 46) asks "How did we become neurochemical selves? How did we come to think about our sadness as a condition called "depression" caused by a chemical imbalance in the brain and amenable to treatment by drugs that would "rebalance" these chemicals? How did we come to experience our worries at home and at work as "generalized anxiety disorder" also caused by a chemical imbalance which can be corrected by drugs?" The influences of "medical neoliberalism" has been pointed out as a key mechanism in modifying discourses around depression and its treatment. The dominance of market rationality have commodified mental health research and practice to extend this rationality to the management of individuals and populations – in this way, the Movement for Global Mental Health have been accused to aid in the expansion of biomedical ideology (Cosgrove & Karter 2018). Attention is drawn from the importance of public policy towards individual-level factors in understanding depression, compounded by reduced spending on services that create supporting environments to combat depression and shifts of responsibility for health status to individuals and their families (Teghtsoonian 2009). The biomedical model of depression allows for these shifts to happen, illustrating the power of discourse (Foucault 1978). Rather than biochemical roots, depression might rather – or at the very least, also – be the result of modern life, insecurity in the labour market, increasing isolation and loneliness, exponential growth in standards to perform, the disappearance of community (J. Moncrieff 2008). Depression is touted as a "disease of modernity", and aspects such as declining social capital; greater inequality and competition; obesity, malnourishment, poor diet and sedentary lifestyle; sleep deprivation and loneliness are very much contributing to depression in contemporary times (Hidaka 2012).

2 The governance of mental health care in South Africa

Introduction

State-provided mental health care during pre-democratic South Africa

To understand mental health care, one needs to understand its structure and position within broader systems and, ideally, in terms of a substantial historical trajectory. It is, after all, a specific way in which societies organise resources in response to a particularly defined social "problem" (for a lack of a better term). In the subject of medical and health care history, mental health care has been a very popular focus. One only has to think of the vast works produced by Roy Porter, Andrew Scull, Anne Harrington and others, that map out how mental illness transformed from a concern for spirituality and religious affliction, to the various biological and psychological models that contend for supremacy in many academic and medical circles today. As noted earlier, the understanding of mental illness is critical, as it becomes the pivot around which services are modelled. Medical historians describe in great detail how shifting understandings of the root causes and nature of mental illness led to the proliferation of particular in vogue models of care such as asylums, surgical intervention, psychoanalysis and deinstitutionalisation. Even though his historical accounts have been called into question (though he is not, nor would call himself, a historian), Michel Foucault contributed a great deal to these insights.

Mental health care trajectories associated with a Western narrative, especially the dominance of psychiatry and the proliferation of asylums during the last two centuries, also emerged in colonial areas. In countries where racial separation was promoted in public as well as in private spaces, institutional care for people with severe mental illness was mixed (for instance, in Australia and South Africa), although there would be racial segregation within institutions. The histories of mental health care in South Africa's colonial period have been covered to a large extent by Sally Swartz, Lynn Gillis, as well as in Tiffany Fawn Jones' *Psychiatry, Mental Institutions, and the Mad in Apartheid South Africa*. These histories largely expand on our knowledge of colonial psychiatry with a focus on the role of asylums, and follow a similar

Table 2.1 Major developments in public mental health care in South Africa

1699–1818	First colonial hospitals built, with facilities for confining and restraining "the mad"
1836	Mentally ill people transferred to Robben Island, along with lepers and chronically ill
1860	Humanist reforms in Robben Island, moving away from mechanical restraints towards different therapies
1876–1897	Several psychiatric hospitals built throughout the British colony in South Africa
1916	Mental Disorders Act No. 38
1920	South African National Council of Mental Health established
1944	Mental institution administration transferred from the Department of Interior to the Department of Public Health
1946	Tara Hospital opens
1953	Tara Hospital initiates the first psychiatric outpatient programme in South Africa
1957	Mental Disorders Amendment Act removes the class of "social defective", changes the name of the Commissioner for Mental Disorder to Commissioner of Mental Hygiene
1963	Smith Mitchell opens its first long-term care institution
1966	Society of Psychiatrists and Neurologists of South Africa formed
1967	Commission of Inquiry to Inquire into the Responsibility of Mentally Deranged Persons and Related Matters (Rumpff Commission)
	Committee of Inquiry into the Care of Mentally Deficient Persons
1972	Commission of Inquiry into the Mental Disorders Act, 1916 (Act No. 38 of 1916, as amended) and Related Matters (Van Wyk Commission)
1978	American Psychiatric Association investigates and reports on Smith Mitchell facilities
1981–1990	Stanley Platman conducts bi-annual reviews of Smith Mitchell facilities
1983	Royal College of Psychiatrists investigates Smith Mitchell facilities
1987	Responsibility for psychiatric hospitals transferred to provincial authority
1994	Racial distinctions among patients abolished
1997	Truth and Reconciliation Commission, Mental Health Workshop held
	White Paper for the Transformation of the Health System, accompanied by Mental Health Policy Guidelines
2002	Mental Health Care Act No. 17
2012	National Mental Health Policy Framework and Strategic Plan 2013–2020
2015–2019	Life Esidimeni events

Sources: Jones 2012; Gillis 2012; Janse van Rensburg 2018.

narrative to Western developments (see a summary in Table 2.1). Accordingly, Dutch and British rulers, during the first two centuries of colonial domination, built asylums in step with European developments in mental health care. At first, these were largely to constrain patients, but later humanist reforms allowed for a broader range of therapies. The British colonial expansion of the late 19th century saw the construction of a number of mental asylums throughout the country. The first half of the 20th century saw the formalisation of South Africa's psychiatric administration, through the promulgation of various acts and the formation of mental health professional bodies. As the country moved closer into systemic and overt racialisation, a close relationship between psychiatry, racism and oppression emerged more pointedly (Swartz 2009).

The Smith Mitchell and Co arrangement

The distinct racialisation of mental health care during pre-democratic South Africa was exposed during the height of apartheid, part of a growing international wave of protest against its inhuman policies. A 1975 editorial in the *Sunday Times* alleged that the apartheid government outsourced psychiatric care for (mostly black) state patients to a private, for-profit company, leading to patterns of woefully subhuman standards of care. This arrangement was in place between 1963 and 1989, where Smith Mitchell and Co – a Johannesburg-based chartered accountancy firm – operated a number of mental health residential facilities, compensated by the government. At the time, senior apartheid cabinet members had financial interests in multiple companies and sectors, of which psychiatric inpatient care was one. Specifically, Connie Mulder (apartheid cabinet minister) and David Tabatznik (chairman of Smith Mitchell and Co), were directors of the Randfontein Non-White Sanatorium (PTY) and Randwest Sanatorium (PTY), positions that Mulder stepped down from but still retained shares in various Smith Mitchell and Co companies (West 1979). The arrangement between the government and Smith Mitchell and Co started in the company providing TB care for black patients, which later turned into psychiatric care provided from reclaimed mining buildings (Ure 2015). Ultimately, Smith Mitchell and Co were granted almost exclusive rights to operate mental institutions in Bantustan and other areas (Jewkes 1984), to the extent that during the 1980s more than 40 percent of the national number of mental health care beds was controlled by the company (Jones 2012)[1].

State patients were transferred from government-run hospitals to 13 Smith Mitchell and Co facilities, and the government had to compensate the company £35.50 for white patients, £18 for coloured patients and £7.50 for black patients (per person, annually). Nine of the 13 facilities were designated non-white, where the standards of care were by far the worst. In these facilities, "care" transcended merely custodial dimensions, to also include labour – thereby mimicking the tendency of the apartheid government to draw profit from black labour. Patients were put to work, Smith Mitchell and Co contracting their services out to other companies, to produce wire hangers, leg guards for the mining sector, and carrier bags (Jones 2012).

Claims of psychiatric malpractice against non-white patients were mounting from the international community, and during the 1977 meeting of the World Psychiatric Association (WPA), members of the American Psychiatric Association (APA) added their voice against the apartheid

Box 2.1 Excerpt from Fleur de Villiers' 1975 depiction of Smith Mitchell and Co facilities in the *Sunday Times* (de Villiers 1975)

One could imagine the following description to be of the Nazi concentration camps ... except for the location and recordkeeping:

The heads were shaved.
Their eyes glazed.
They walked around with seedy, broken work uniforms and bare feet.
There were thousands of them, like children.
They belonged to the group of mental patients held in the condemned mine barracks
The records were not openly available and filled with inaccurate notes.
The number of these human warehouses where care is reduced to a minimum and cure a forgotten word is growing year by year – as are the profits of the company which now has such a monopoly on madness that as one authority told me, "it can virtually dictate mental health care in South Africa".

government, as part of a growing criticism by the World Health Organization, the Church of Scientology, the foreign and local press. The South African government denied that psychiatric institutionalisation was used for anything apart from medical reasons, and under increasing outside pressure, the government offered a formal invitation to the APA to inspect Smith Mitchell and Co facilities. The delegation included Jeanne Spurlock, Jack Weinberg and Charles Pinderhughes, and was led by Harvard University psychiatric ethics expert Alan Stone (American Psychiatric Association 1979).

Following a period of negotiation over the terms of the visit, the delegation proceeded to investigate the following claims:

1. An unacceptable mortality rate among patients
2. Substandard levels of care
3. Abusive practices
4. Grossly inadequate professional staff
5. Inappropriate use of electroconvulsive therapy and psychopharmaceutical drugs
6. Exploitation of patients as labour source
7. Psychiatric confinement of political dissidents
8. Apartheid causes mental health harm

The basic standards of judging these claims relied on the questions whether medical and psychiatric care was insufficient to the extent that patient well-being was hindered, and how the standards of treatment and care of black patients compared with that of white patients. By these standards, the committee found cause for concern – especially in terms of avoidable deaths, substandard care, abusive practices, inadequate medical staff, and the destructive effects of apartheid on mental health. Predictably, the blame for negative outcomes were moved from the apartheid state to Smith Mitchell and Co as service providers, though the report admirably focused on systemic causes rather than on agential (American Psychiatric Association 1979). The following conclusion was reached:

> The Smith Mitchell facilities can be viewed as only a subsystem of the larger South African apartheid system, reflecting in microcosm some of its pathogenic governmental and social structures and processes. A powerful contrived reality has been developed in South Africa that favors and protects whites while excluding, neglecting, or oppressing blacks. Smith Mitchell functions in this context – indeed, probably would not exist without it – and must conform to it.
>
> (American Psychiatric Association 1979, 1506)

The APA investigation was followed up by a report, "The Case for South Africa's Expulsion from International Psychiatry", penned by Rachel Jewkes for the United Nations Centre against Apartheid (Jewkes 1984). Commenting on the apartheid government's response to the APA report, she underlined their "racist arrogance and contempt for the lives of black South Africans", citing their official responses to critiques of substandard care:

> Black patients are not provided with beds and have to sleep on the floors because "like so many other Africans ... they prefer to sleep that way". There is no toilet paper for the black patients because "when toilet paper is provided in hospitals (the patients) misuse it, causing sewerage blockages and inconvenience to their fellow patients". And there are no shoes for black patients because they "sell their shoes", "prefer to go without them" and "would kick their fellow patients".
>
> (Jewkes 1984, 4)

The main critique of this report was that psychiatry has been reduced to a political tool, used to repress political opposition and promote the key tenets of apartheid ideology – particularly its primary motive of cheap black labour. Importantly, apartheid definitions of mental illness allowed for the involuntary institutionalisation of black people who are perceived to not see the necessity of apartheid ideology, non-observance of specific laws constituted mental ill-health that required state intervention (Jewkes 1984).

The Smith Mitchell and Co arrangement was but one feature of mental health care during apartheid, but a telling one. The state was in charge of providing mental health care to the public, but put in place draconian policies to disaggregate the public according to race, which accordingly allowed for the investment into some and the disinvestment in others. Black psychiatric inpatients' extreme vulnerability did not absolve them from also being harnessed in the massive labour machinery put in place to fuel the apartheid system and help retain power; the parallels to slavery are obvious. Importantly, the mental health professions – especially psychiatry – legitimised this exploitation, and underlines how deeply engrained the apartheid ideology was. Psychiatry often shadowed government policy by putting in place practices with racist effects. These included inadequate provision of accommodation for the black insane in colonial asylums, discriminatory treatment regimes in which the white insane had better care than their black counterparts, and scientific justifications for patterns of diagnosis that treated black and white patients as biologically different groups (Swartz, 1995a and 1995b). This distinction was abolished – formally and officially at least – when South Africa achieved democracy in 1994, opening up a new chapter (or rather, a new book altogether) in South Africa's mental health care trajectory.

Public mental health care in post-apartheid South Africa

Towards a democratic public health system

Reforms in South Africa's public mental health system during the first few years after democracy were substantially tied to wide-scale attempts to transform the health system from its racist, colonial roots to an equitable, accessible and efficient system built on the principles of primary health care. The newly elected ANC government had a mammoth task on hand – to transform the health system in such a way to deliver on the hope pinned on their decades of struggle for equity. The country's first democratic government inherited a population made up largely of an impoverished black population, living in contexts of overcrowding, poor sanitation, malnutrition, a high degree of stress, not to mention a debilitating sense of injustice. The result was extraordinary levels of poverty-related illness, with very little access to formal health services (Coovadia, Jewkes, Barron, Sanders, & McIntyre 2009a; H. Van Rensburg & Engelbrecht 2012b). David Harrison (2009a) provided a well-crafted summary of this period, noting that the new dispensation was under pressure to demonstrate rapid improvements in health system outcomes, while also "addressing the intractable health management issues that bedevil efficiency and drive up costs". The largest and probably most important innovation during this time was the introduction of a district-based system of care, very much based on the ANC's National Health Plan and the PHC principles of the Alma Ata Declaration, which decentralised service delivery to local areas according to primary, secondary and tertiary levels of care. Country territories – including the 14 Bantustans – were unified into a national health department, delegating power to nine provincial departments (Coovadia et al. 2009a). Key legislation and policy were introduced, including free PHC, an essential drugs programme, legislation providing choice on the termination of pregnancy and targeted tobacco use prevention. There was a revitalisation of hospitals, expansion and improvement of clinics (1,345 new clinics were built and 263 upgraded), improved population immunization and improved equity in health expenditure among districts (Harrison 2009a; H. Van Rensburg & Engelbrecht 2012b). Despite admirable progress – including the wide-scale improvement of access to housing, sanitation, and electricity supply, and the roll-out of a massive welfare programme to support 12.4 million people in need by 2008 – several critical missteps led to substantial losses in South Africa's development goals. Under the now infamous Mbeki regime, privatisation and neoliberal-inspired policy allowed for increasing inequality. The government's AIDS denialism during this time was particularly damaging, with estimations of 330 000 lives lost and 35 000 babies born with HIV due to the government's refusal to provide life-saving ARV's to the public sector (Chigwedere, Seage, Gruskin, Lee, & Essex 2008). The knock-on effects of this strategy on other health conditions (such as TB and hypertension), on the capacity of the health system, not to mention on wider society (upsetting family and community dynamics, entrenching poverty, stigma and fear) are arguably still felt in many communities, and will take generations to correct. The damage of this period has been mitigated somewhat by iterations of the HIV & AIDS and STI Strategic Plan for South Africa, as well as the roll-out of the world's largest public ARV programme. Nonetheless, poor stewardship led to a lack of community involvement in health service provisioning, and insufficient local political accountability hamstrung the ideals of the National Health Act (Coovadia et al. 2009a). Mismanagement and political interference and corruption in many instances led to supply chain bottlenecks, hospital and clinic disrepair, and widespread dissatisfaction among the health workforce with work conditions (H. Van Rensburg & Engelbrecht 2012b).

Following Mbeki's rule, a renewed effort was applied by the government to promote a unified health system that responds to the ideals of universal health coverage. Nevertheless, government efforts to initiate effective reform were severely constrained by critical health system challenges, the most pressing of which were categorised by Harrison (2009a) as a failure to prevent and control epidemics, inequitable allocation and distribution of financial and human resources, and challenges related to health systems management. Specifically, in the period 2010–2015, this included the prevention and treatment of HIV/AIDS, TB and DR-TB, and alcohol abuse; unequal patterns in financing and spending between provinces and levels of care, as well as in the distribution of human resources for health; and poor quality of care and operational efficiency, inadequate devolution of authority, poor health worker morale, and a lack of leadership and innovation (especially on provincial level) (Harrison 2009a). These afflictions continue to haunt the South African health system, and the introduction of National Health Insurance has often been framed as a panacea to overcome these deficiencies. Reform was made tangible by introducing a Green and White Paper for National Health Insurance, tabling a National Health Insurance Act in parliament, and introducing a strategy to revitalise PHC. A growing narrative during these developments, especially under Dr Aaron Motsoaledi's direction, was that the powerful private health sector is a major blockage in the path to universal health coverage in South Africa's health system. The prevailing discourse was one of socialist ideals in health care versus liberal, free market conceptions – very much mirroring the heated nature of debates surrounding Barack Obama's introduction of the Patient Protection and Affordable Care Act of 2010 in the United States during the same period.

Private sector growth

During the 1990s, South Africa saw an almost unbridled expansion of privatised health care (Development Bank of Southern Africa 2008; Harrison 2009a). The South African health system allows for the operations of non-state, for-profit health care providers, under the legislative sovereignty of the state. This includes, among others, hospital groups, individual, and group medical practices (Janse van Rensburg et al. 2018). The growth in this sector was exemplified by expenditure per head on medical schemes increasing to triple that of public health expenditure in 1996, increasing further to six times in 2006; almost three-quarters of general practitioners (a vital part of district PHC) worked in the private sector by the end of the 1990s (Coovadia et al. 2009a). Taking advantage from an increasingly enabling climate, private hospital groups took a firm foothold in the developing South African health system. From 25 hospitals and 2,346 beds in 1976, to 101 hospitals and 10,936 beds in 1989, to 216 hospitals and 31,067 beds in 2010 (by comparison, the public sector had 410 hospitals and 88,920 beds in 2010) (Van den Heever 2012), the private hospital sector is an incredibly powerful network in post-apartheid South Africa. By 2017, 524 private for-profit health care facilities were counted, with 40,514 licenced beds – this included day clinics, drug and alcohol rehabilitation, and mental health institutions (Econex 2017). Three of the largest groups – Mediclinic, Netcare and Life Health care – expanded to the extent that they extended their capital to other countries and regions, on top of being listed on several stock exchange markets. By 2016, private hospitals contributed to 1.3% of gross domestic product (GDP), an amount of R55.5 bn; it generated R16.4 bn tax revenue; sustained R144.1 bn of capital stock (Econex 2017). This growth can be partly explained by corporate capital (especially in the mining sector), as well as by an increasing neoliberal tone in South Africa's macroeconomic landscape into the 2000s – the result has been a political economy with much stronger private influence than in other low-and-middle income countries (Coovadia et al. 2009a; Bongani M. Mayosi & Benatar 2014).

The role of the non-profit sector

South African CSOs have been given a "light touch" by the state compared to other LMIC settings – no doubt as part of a firm move away from an apartheid history of strict CSO control (Batley 2006). By implementing the Non-profit Organisations Act (71 of 1997), instituting a voluntary registration system, and by creating a Directorate for Non-profit Organisations, the post-apartheid government moved swiftly to create a fiscal, legal and political environment conducive to collaboration between the state and CSOs. This environment created new opportunities for CSOs, especially elevating their service delivery role (often to the detriment of their role as activists and government accountability regulators) (Habib 2005). CSOs either became part of business networks or tendered for government and transnational funding (Habib & Taylor 1999). Shifts towards democratisation almost inevitably challenge the legitimacy and capacity of CSOs to serve as "pseudo-democratic representatives of the poor", undermining broader democratic norms (Mitlin, Hickey, & Bebbington 2007).

The role of CSOs as community stewards has further been challenged by global forces. The Paris Declaration on Aid Effectiveness and the Accra Agenda for Action significantly altered the ways in which global funding flows towards CSOs, importantly funnelling funding through national government infrastructure (Organisation for Economic Cooperation and Development 2008). This development was designed to enhance country ownership, donor priority alignment and harmonisation, impact measurement and improved mutual accountability (a type of global governance of the neoliberal governmentality kind) (André Janse van Rensburg et al. 2018). Nevertheless, the global funding environment of the mid-2000s – spurred on by an intractable AIDS pandemic – restructured the relationship between the state and CSOs, one where CSO independence was curtailed towards a co-option into the role of state service provider (Birdsall & Kelly 2007). In contemporary South Africa, CSOs have often picked up the reigns of service delivery where it was dropped by government, and there is a heavy reliance in some sectors on CSO-delivered services – this includes social and welfare services, health promotion and prevention services in clinics and schools, substance abuse and prevention, and the provisioning of residential and day care services for vulnerable populations.

Mental health care's post-apartheid journey

How did mental health care fit into this wide-sweeping narrative? Admirably, mental health was prioritised from the very start of reform, having a central place in what would become a key guiding document for South Africa's health system reconfiguration – the ANC's National Health Plan for South Africa (World Health Organization, African National Congress, & United Nations Children's Fund 1994). It stressed the notion of mental health *and* well-being, describing causes of mental ill health to include materials and social conditions as well as other health and well-being conditions. With a central focus on eliminating service fragmentation by adopting integration strategies, the document was ahead of its time, calling for "a multi-sectoral and integrated approach to mental health service", which includes the integration of mental health services into different sectors such as general health care, welfare and education systems. It endorsed the development of multi-level inter-sectoral structures from which mental health care should be co-ordinated among different government departments as well as all relevant levels of service provision. Community care and support services for PLWMI was a prominent feature, and the document called for the "development of non-governmental community-based mental health care services and fostering cooperation between the various mental health service providers", including increased cooperation with traditional healers (World Health Organization, African National Congress, & United Nations Children's Fund 1994). These messages would echo throughout the next 25 years, and repeated in South Africa's National Mental Health Policy Framework and Strategic Plan 2013–2020 (National Department of Health 2013).

The tone of the ANC Health Plan was continued in the White Paper for the Transformation of the Health System in South Africa (National Department of Health 1997), meant as a roadmap for national, provincial and district health system restructuring. It furthered the directive that health services should be provided in an integrated manner across different sectors, calling for collaboration in care between governmental, non-governmental and private services. A dedicated chapter on mental health care outlined the provision of "a comprehensive and community-based mental health and related services ... planned and co-ordinated at national, provincial, district and community levels, and integrated with other health services" (chapter 12). Inter-sectoral collaboration was to be co-ordinated at national level, planned and facilitated at provincial level, and maintained at district and community levels. Role-players included CSOs, private for-profit practitioners, and traditional healers.

An intention to increase access to mental health care was rooted in The Primary Health Care Package for South Africa (National Department of Health 2000) and in A District Hospital Service Package for South Africa (National Department of Health 2002). A core overarching standard in both documents relate to collaboration, calling on facilities to collaborate with relevant public entities as well as with civil society and workplaces in catchment areas of health facilities. Regarding mental health care, such facilities should be acquainted with community support and referral organisations, and should seek out collaborative relationships with traditional healers, religious, and non-governmental community services and groups. These initiatives were transferred to a first dedicated mental health policy – the Policy Guidelines on Child and Adolescent Mental Health (National Department of Health 2003). This document framed mental health services for children and adolescents according to national, provincial and district levels within a PHC, intersectoral approach. Again, it stressed the need for collaboration and integration across government departments, CSOs, community structures and families. The main focus of the policy fell on providing a supportive external environment, information sharing, skills-building, counselling and service accessibility.

During this time, one of the most important developments happened for mental health care reform, namely the introduction of the Mental Health Care Act (17 of 2002) (MHCA) (South African Government 2002). The MHCA was a firm step away from the restrictive apartheid-era Mental Health Act No. 18 of 1973, with a concern for community safety overriding concerns for human rights. In terms of health systems structure, the previous act also framed psychiatric care as separate from general health services. General practitioners were not required to provide mental health services, and mental health care were very much centralised in large, urban psychiatric hospitals, with little to no care in rural areas and communities (Burns 2008). The MHCA rode on the wave of human rights driven by the country's widely applauded Constitution. People with mental illness were designated as "users", moving away from the custodial term of "patients". In addition to treatment, services were also to include rehabilitation and recovery, and mental health care was to be fully integrated into general health services, especially by extending its human resource body to include general practitioners, collaboration with private for-profit and non-profit sectors including with traditional healers. This directive was further supported by the National Health Act (61 of 2003), which obliges the DoH to establish co-ordinated relationships between public and private service providers, and allows for formal agreements between government departments and municipalities, and "any private practitioner, private health establishment or non-governmental organisation" (Section 45) (South African Government 2004).

The MHCA continued to dictate that, in line with PHC principles, people should have access to mental health care close to where they live, and PHC integration would become a major focus of future reforms. This includes providing primary mental health care at PHC facilities, district hospitals and in community settings. An important feature in the MHCA was the introduction of 72-hour observation measures, where people suffering from acute psychiatric conditions (for instance, violent drug-induced psychosis) could be involuntarily admitted to a designated hospital for a 72-hour period of observation. Following a review by clinicians and the mental health review board, the service user could be referred for further in-hospital care, or discharged for outpatient treatment. There was a strong shift in acknowledging and promoting the human rights and ability to appeal of service users, overseen by mental health review boards that were to be established as independent ombud (South African Government 2002). The MHCA provided a legally-mandated catalyst for change, but whole-scale mental health reform suffered from the act's assumption that the three-tiered health system was ready and accepting of mental health services: "While the Act proclaims, reality dictates" (Szabo & Kaliski 2017). Mental health care at PHC and community levels were still very much undeveloped, despite attempts to initiate reform. Indeed, early on, Petersen (2000) pertinently asked whether comprehensive, integrated mental health care in South Africa would be achievable given serious barriers in PHC facilities. It became apparent that, despite these early policy gains, mental health care still had a long way to go.

Following the initial period of policy and legislative reform after achieving democracy, South Africa had to achieve the lofty ideals set in the Mandela era. Critically important research would be conducted during this stage. The South African Stress and Health (SASH) survey, in line with the World Mental Health Survey (WMHS), was conducted between 2003 and 2004, and, at the time of writing, remains the only nationally representative epidemiological database of mental disorders in South Africa. The many publications emanating from this survey would become a staple in publications, especially in journal papers, and informed policy on a national level. By being part of the WMHS, SASH also allowed for comparisons of mental health data with other countries (Stein, Williams, & Kessler 2009). During this period, a group of researchers collaborated with the DoH and the WHO to describe public sector mental health bed/facility ratios (Lund, Flisher, Porteus, & Lee 2002); develop norms and standards for mental health care (Lund & Flisher 2006); mental health indicators on hospital and community level (Lund & Flisher 2003); and process indicators to monitor and evaluate public sector mental health services (Lund & Flisher 2001). These inputs provided an evidence base for mental health service delivery and evaluation and were important bricks in the construction of the mental health care wall.

Global mental health and subsequent explosion in research

On the heels of these baseline developments, there followed what would become a central development in mental health care reform globally, namely the Movement for Global Mental Health was launched. The Movement would catalyse funding for a series of studies that would become the pivot around future mental health care reform, and included local researchers that were deeply embedded in the drive towards the development of mental health care beyond hospitals. This included leaders in the emerging field of public mental health, people like Alan Flisher, Crick Lund, Inge Petersen, Arvin Bhana, Lesley Swartz and Soraya Seedat (among others), and included a host of new students in what would become known as "Global Mental Health". Perhaps officially launched by the 2007 Lancet series for Global Mental Health (Lancet Global Mental Health Group 2007), the Movement for Global Mental Health helped lobbying efforts for increased funding towards mental health system strengthening in LMICs. In South Africa, this led to a series of key studies: Mental Health and Poverty Project (MHaPP) 2005–2010; Programme for Improving Mental Health Care (PRIME) 2011–2019; Comorbid Affective

Disorders, AIDS/HIV, and Long Term Health (COBALT) 2013–2018; Emerging Mental Health Systems in Low- and Middle-Income Countries (EMERALD) 2012–2017; and Africa Focus on Intervention Research for Mental Health (AFFIRM) 2011–2016[2]. Though different in scope and aim, these studies sought to provide evidence on how the principles of integrated primary mental health care can be achieved on the ground, a science-driven response to calls from the policy and legislative spheres.

Despite increased global and local attention to the ideals of public mental health as part of universal health coverage, South Africa conspicuously still lacked a national policy, a document that can help guide provincial governments to put in place key structures and processes to promote comprehensive, integrated mental health care. A key moment after the initial Global Mental Health surge in South Africa was a National Mental Health Summit in 2012, the culmination of provincial summits held prior to capture local inputs into the state of mental health care. Attended by government departments, CSOs, the WHO, academic institutions, research organisations, professional bodies, traditional healers, health professionals and advocacy and user groups. The Minister of Health at the time, Dr Aaron Motsoaledi, remarked in his opening statement at the event that "I am sure that you will agree with me that this summit must represent a departure from mental health being considered a Cinderella of the health system!" (National Department of Health 2012b). In essence, as illustrated in Box 2.2, the minister officially endorsed mental health as a priority programme in South Africa's health system reform trajectory, and called for tangible future steps to affirm this emphasis.

Employing the strategic theme "Scaling up investment in mental health for a long and healthy life for all South Africans", the Summit generated and adopted the Ekurhuleni Declaration on Mental Health (National Mental Health Summit 2012). The Declaration re-affirmed the centrality of PHC principles as compass for reform and highlighted integrated mental health care as a principle mechanism with which to achieve efficient and equitable health services. The Declaration also underlined mental health's position within broader reforms, stating that it has to form part of National Health Insurance and related programmes. Sixteen interim goals, and 11 longer-term goals were outlined, among which the finalisation of the draft Mental Health Policy Framework was probably the most pressing (National Mental Health Summit 2012).

National policy

The adoption of the Comprehensive Mental Health Action Plan 2013–2020 by the World Health Assembly in 2013 set the stage for the introduction of South Africa's first formal mental health policy, the National Mental Health Policy Framework and Strategic Plan 2013–2020 (MHPF) (National Department of Health 2013), formally adopted by the National Health

Box 2.2 Excerpt from the Minister of Health's speech at the 2012 National Mental Health Summit

I believe this summit represents a significant milestone for mental health in this country. In this regard we must collectively make maximum use of this opportunity and provide both evidence-based inputs as well as personal experiences to ensure that the objectives of this summit are realised. This summit must:

(a) review both the quality and quantity of mental health services that we currently provide;
(b) identify the key challenges in the mental health care system;
(c) provide information on best practices that have emerged since 1994; and
(d) agree on key interventions that must be prioritised and implemented as we reorganise and strengthen the health system.

Over the two days we must deliberate and propose a road map for mental health as this area of work is central to the achievement of the outcome of "a long and healthy life for all South Africans".

Council in July 2013 (Stein 2014). In step with the country's more participatory post-apartheid policy-making procedures, the Policy was informed by the provincial consultative process for the National Mental Health Summit. It also was informed by a literature and policy review; a situation analysis including key informant interviews; and alignment with DoH and WHO strategy. The MHPF was also explicitly aligned with the White Paper for the Transformation of the Health System, as well as national norms for people with severe psychiatric conditions, community-based mental health care, and child and adolescent mental health services, and standards for mental health care in South Africa (Stein 2014). The MHPF detailed roles and responsibilities for mental health care stakeholders, in line with the Constitution and the National Health Act. This included mandates for the Minister of Health; Members of Executive Councils (MECs), Health managers at national and provincial levels; the National Health Council; Provincial Health Councils and District Health Councils. The vision, mission, objectives and 12 action points (see Table 2.2) speak to a comprehensive overhaul of the mental health system, with ambitious goals that echo the original intent of the ANC Health Plan (National Department of Health 2013).

There is no doubt that the MHPF was an instrumental piece of policy, an embodiment of the optimism of the Movement for Global Mental Health as well as of South Africa's determined struggle for a health system that matches Mandela's ideals of equity and social justice. Now that the MHPF has

Table 2.2 Outlines of the National Mental Health Policy Framework and Strategic Plan 2013–2020

Vision	
Improved mental health for all in South Africa by 2020.	
Mission	
From infancy to old age, the mental health and well-being of all South Africans will be enabled, through the provision of evidence-based, affordable and effective promotion, prevention, treatment and rehabilitation interventions. In partnerships between providers, users, carers and communities, the human rights of people with mental illness will be upheld; they will be provided with care and support; and they will be integrated into normal community life.	
Objectives	
To scale up decentralised integrated primary mental health services, which include community-based care, PHC clinic care, and district hospital level care	
To increase public awareness regarding mental health and reduce stigma and discrimination associated with mental illness	
To promote the mental health of the South African population, through collaboration between the Department of Health and other sectors	
To empower local communities, especially mental health service users and carers, to participate in promoting mental well-being and recovery within their community	
To promote and protect the human rights of people living with mental illness	
To adopt a multi-sectoral approach to tackling the vicious cycle of poverty and mental ill-health	
To establish a monitoring and evaluation system for mental health care	
To ensure that the planning and provision of mental health services is evidence-based	
Areas of action	
1. Organisation of services (according to Community mental health services; The district mental health system; Psychiatric services in general hospitals; and Specialised psychiatric hospitals)	2. Financing
3. Promotion and prevention	4. Inter-sectoral collaboration
5. Advocacy	6. Human rights
7. Special populations	8. Monitoring and evaluation
9. Quality improvement	10. Human resources and training
11. Psychotropic medication	12. Research and evaluation of policy and services

Source: National Department of Health, 2013.

completed its policy cycle, we will need to critically appraise its wins and losses. The MHPF itself was a major win in mental health care reform, the result of cohesive leadership by an influential global network of individual actors and the political commitment provided by global health governance institutions (Stein 2014; Tomlinson & Lund 2012). A comprehensive evaluation still needs to be done of the MHPF, a robust appreciation of the complexities that vexed its implementation. However, the development of one of its core aims – developing a community mental health system – was brutally opened up for scrutiny and critique when the notorious Life Esidimeni events unfolded in 2015–2018, a quintessential discursive event in South Africa's post-apartheid journey in mental health care reform. It would kick off a period of introspection, political blame, and discourses and responsibility, justice and the ethics of care – not to mention the financing of mental health care. However, during the same time, South Africa's globally recognised public mental health academics continued with attempts to translate the content of the MHPF into practice – whereas the period before the MHPF mostly focused on exploring barriers, facilitators and opportunities for public mental health care (especially integrating mental health into PHC platforms and programmes), more recently there seemed to be a more pragmatic shift towards collaborating closely with provincial DoH directorates to implement integrated mental health strategies. The lessons learned during the previous decade needed to be put into practice. Examples here include Screening, brief intervention, and referral to treatment (SBIRT) for risky substance use (van der Westhuizen et al. 2019); the roll-out of monitoring of assertive community interventions to assist people with severe mental disorders (Botha, Koen, Galal, Jordaan, & Niehaus 2014); and the integration of mental health counselling and referral through task-sharing in PHC facilities, using the MhINT model of integration (Petersen, van Rensburg, Gigaba, Luvuno, & Fairall 2020). In many ways though, there is a new horizon for mental health care – the next national policy cycle needs to be developed; there will need to be a close examination of the ways in which mental health care will feature in South Africa's roll-out of National Health Insurance; and, most worryingly, it remains to be seen how the COVID-19 pandemic will alter the health systems landscape. In these early phases, the research, financing and development dimensions of health care have already been irrevocably been changed, and it remains to be seen what this means for mental health care reform.

Civil society

The journey described thus far has been penned largely by the health sector, with little input or action from other relevant sectors. Despite the significant and substantial contributions of civil society to public mental health care, social development, with its stewardship role of the welfare dimensions of the vulnerable in South African communities, have been distressingly silent in descriptions of South Africa's mental health care system. This, of course, means that the role of CSOs and social workers, faith-based actors and support groups have been side-lined in the quest to develop mental health services in health care facilities. Collectively, these "third sector" actors (behind government and business) are known as civil society, a loosely bounded group consisting of "*the wide array of non-governmental and not for profit organizations that have a presence in public life, express the interests and values of their members and others, based on ethical, cultural, political, scientific, religious or philanthropic considerations*" (World Bank, 2020).

A large part of contemporary South African organised civil society – we can refer to this as civil society organisations (CSOs) – has its roots in female-driven Afrikaner nationalist movements that sprung during the first half of the 20th century. After the ravages of the Second Boer War, the Zuid-Afrikaansche Christelijke Vrouevereniging (ACVV) was born, laying the foundations for provincial welfare societies such as the Suid-Afrikaanse Vrouefederasie (SAVF) in Transvaal, the Orangia-Vrouevereniging in the Free State, and the Natalse Christelike Vrouevereniging. These organisations were, on the one hand, an extension of Afrikaner identity-making, the development of a puritan nation rooted in the Dutch Reformed Church and Afrikaner women as mothers of this nation (Du Toit 1996). Philanthropy became a means rather than an end, with a strong focus on the upliftment of poor whites through an evangelical type of welfare, backed by the substantial economic and cultural capital imbued through the Dutch Reformed Church. The myopic focus on white upliftment was abandoned post-1994, but the architecture of these SAVF networks remained, adapting to the democratic transition by adopting a welfare service delivery role for broader society. This narrative is one of many others though, and there are countless (almost quite literally – cannot be counted) CSOs woven into the fabric of South Africa's contemporary welfare landscape.

As South Africa matured as a democracy, its welfare and social services civil society landscape started to organise in a more collective way. Many of the larger organisations formed strategic coalitions to increase their lobbying and influencing power in dealing with the Department of Social Development. This includes the Council for Church Social Services, the National Coalition for Social Services (NACOSS), and the National Association of Welfare Organisations and Non-Governmental Organisations (NAWONGO). NAWONGO would especially become part of a key development in the relationship between state and civil society, with important consequences for mental health service provisioning and funding.

The substantial CSO workforce were formally harnessed by the new ANC government by introducing the Non-profit Organisations Act, 1997 (South African Government 1997b). The purpose of this Act was to provide an environment where strategic partnerships between government and CSOs could be facilitated towards reaching strategic goals. It established an administrative and regulatory framework for CSO activities by establishing the Directorate for Non-profit Organisations within the Department of Social Development. This structure manages the registration and regulation of CSOs according to predetermined strategic actions required in different provinces, in different sectors (South African Government 1997b).

The Mental Health Care Act (17 of 2002) allowed for agreements between national and provincial departments with CSOs, as well as with private for-profit services, as well as for the "authorisation and licensing of health establishments administered under the auspices of State, a non-governmental organisation or private body providing mental health care, treatment and rehabilitation services and conditions to be attached to such authorisation or licence" (South African Government 2002). These directives were further entrenched by the National Health Act (61 of 2003), which instructed the Minister of Health to develop mechanisms that enable co-ordinated relationships between public health services and non-governmental actors, and allowed for public-private partnerships and other agreements between government and non-governmental service providers (South African Government 2004). Collaboration between government and non-government role-players was adopted in the Ekurhuleni Declaration on Mental Health, which was included in the National Mental Health Policy Framework and Strategic Plan 2013–2020 (National Department of Health 2013). This sets the stage further for future mental health system reform, including a focus on inter-sectoral collaboration. More specifically, it provides for the future expansion of community mental health care to formally include CSOs, voluntary groups and consumer organisations. Further, it underlines the responsibility of provincial government to encourage different service collaborations with CSOs.

The devolution of power to provincial governments to come up with strategies to collaborate with non-government actors to provide public mental health care has led to substantial inequalities in how much resources are invested in mental health services, and what output are generated (Lund, Kleintjes, Kakuma, & Flisher 2010). A lack of strategic stewardship from provinces has resulted – in part, at least – in wide variation in the types, sizes and focus of CSOs providing mental health care. In the relative absence of psychiatrists, psychologists and mental health nurses generally and particularly in the public sector, CSOs such as professional organisations, religious groups, patient support groups, and traditional healers have significantly contributed to mental, emotional, and spiritual well-being in poor communities (Wolvaardt et al. 2008). Much like in other countries, CSOs have been especially instrumental in the provision of residential/institutionalisation services for people living with mental illness (World Health Organization 2008). CSOs further act as liaison between families and government agencies for grant access, by providing material support to families waiting for grant application processing and catalysing government action in expediting application processes (Rosenberg et al. 2008). Importantly, by often representing and servicing citizens without voice, CSOs fulfil a central democratic role by focusing their efforts on specific individuals and groups who have been rendered vulnerable by broader society.

Perhaps the most important role of CSOs in South Africa's mental health system is filling the gaps in non-facility based, community-based care. South Africa spends approximately R8.37 bn, 5% of its annual health budget, on inpatient and outpatient mental health care, that includes R250.2 m in transfers to contracted CSOs, across all provinces. This amounts to R180.90 per uninsured person, of which approximately R12.30 is paid towards transfers to contracted CSOs (Docrat, Lund, & Besada 2019). This suggests that the vast majority of the health budget does not follow people to community settings but remains concentrated in biomedical institutions. The path dependency of institutionalised-heavy mental health systems seems to be a global feature of reform – there are not many examples globally of successful transition from asylum-focused to community-focused mental health systems. There are, of course, examples. In high-income settings with relatively large resources in mental health professional capacity, there has been strides in changing the locus of care to people's home spheres. In Belgian municipalities, multidisciplinary mobile crisis teams affiliated with non-governmental hospitals map out and monitor people with severe mental conditions, with intensive home visits for following acute psychiatric events to prevent suicidal behaviour, promote healthy living behaviours and prevent re-admission and further harm (Santermans, Zeeuws, Vanderbruggen, & Crunelle 2019). In Quebec, Canada, the Quebec Mental Health Reform programme promoted the development of integrated service networks, which includes collaboration and coordination between local community community centres, CSOs, private medical clinics and other relevant inter-sectoral resources (Fleury et al. 2016). This has also been demonstrated in the better resourced Western Cape, where assertive community interventions have been championed as a mechanism to reduce the gaps between communities and specialised hospitals (Botha, Koen, Ushma, Jordaan, & Niehaus 2014).

Contemporary mental health system

We have briefly considered the three groups of actors involved in the mental health system in contemporary South Africa. However, identifying actors is one thing, but getting a sense of a system in its structural sense requires mapping out their activities in terms of relationships with each other. The diagram in Figure 2.1 is an illustrated attempt to make sense of these complexities, and provides a map to better understand the political dimensions involved in mental health care in South Africa. The diagram is informed by different studies describing mental health care, especially from a national/provincial perspective (Lund et al., 2010; Lund, Petersen, Kleintjes, & Bhana 2012; Lund, Petersen, Kleintjes, & Bhana 2012; Petersen & Lund 2011), as well as district-level configurations in different areas in the country (Janse van Rensburg, Petersen, et al. 2018; Mkize et al. 2004; Mkize & Uys 2004; Robertson & Szabo 2017). Finally, this is an attempt to encapsulate what actually happens on the ground, in distinction to what is supposed to happen as mandated. The ideal configuration as mapped out in the MHPF, the Mental Health care Act 2002 and in other related strategy documents are therefore not entirely covered. For instance, as part of South Africa's PHC

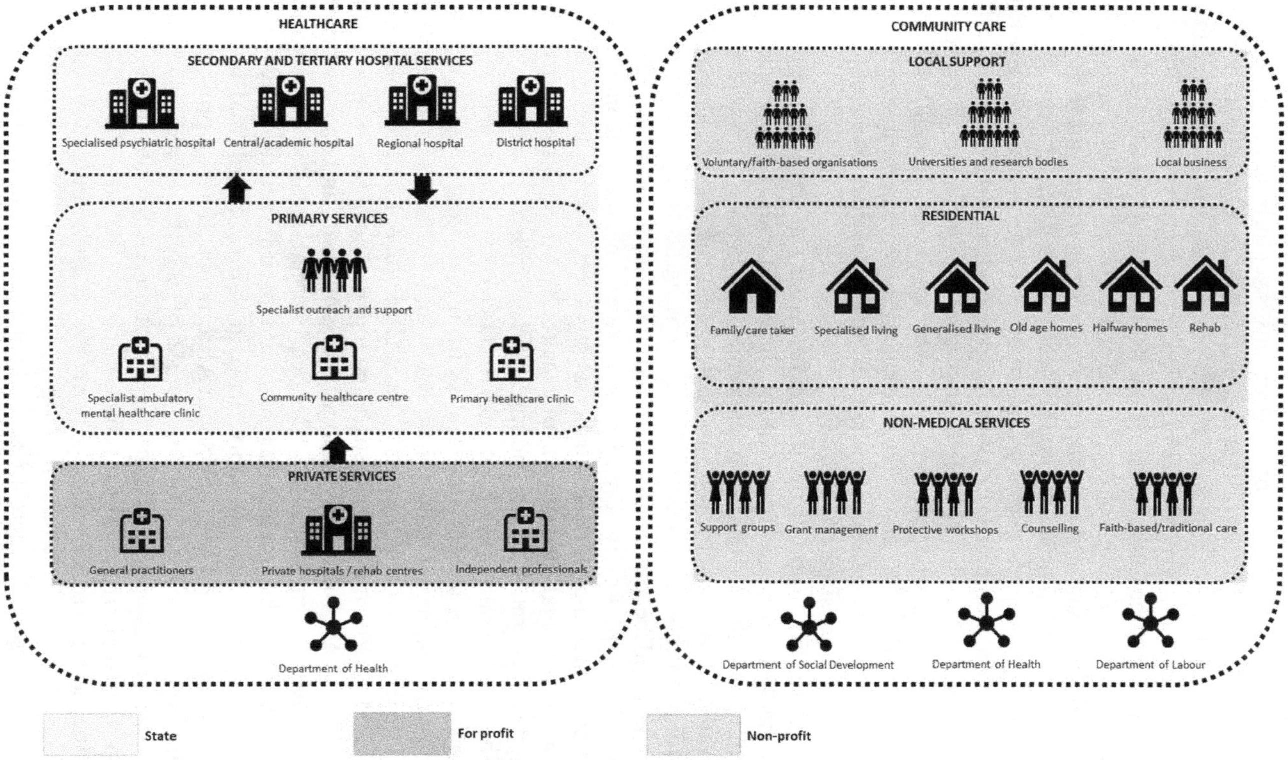

Figure 2.1 Structure of mental health care in contemporary South Africa.
Source: Author.

Re-engineering initiative, ward-based outreach teams are supposed to conduct household screening of all households and refer as required. However, after approximately eight years of roll-out, this is yet to be in place at scale.

The crux of this illustration is that mental health care is significantly tied to place; in this way, services consist of health care, largely provided in facilities, and a range of non-medical services provided in community settings. In South Africa's three-tiered health system, mental health care is provided at tertiary, secondary and primary levels of care (Lund et al. 2012). On PHC level, people with severe mental illness mainly receive symptom management in the form of dispensing follow-up medication. People who have suffered from acute or chronic symptoms, such as psychosis, are often sent back home after a period of hospitalisation, where they are tied to a specific clinic where they can fetch their medicine. Although PHC clinic staff need to also monitor comorbid conditions among this population, staff shortages, lack of skills and persistent stigma render PHC clinic-based care as mostly medicine dispensing. In acute cases, the clinic can also refer clients to hospitals where more specialised human resources are situated.

Although district hospitals are designated as part of the PHC system, in terms of mental health care district hospitals are deemed a secondary level of care (Lund et al. 2012). Here, a critical dimension of care for severe mental illness is the 72-hour emergency observation mandate for district hospitals. A According to this directive, people experiencing acute and severe mental symptoms should be kept in isolation and under observation for 72 hours. The Mental Health Review Board should determine the outcome of this observation, which may include further observation, referral for more care, or discharge (National Department of Health 2012a). This mechanism has not operated very well thus far, and the abilities of district hospitals to provide 72-hour observation has been substantially marred by a lack of isolation infrastructure, a lack of staff and skills in managing severe symptoms such as psychosis, high administrative loads, and low levels of engagement with review boards (Docrat, Besada, Cleary, Daviaud, & Lund 2019; Ramlall, Chipps, & Mars 2010). In some district and regional hospitals, mental health outpatient units are run by psychologists, psychiatrists, and social workers, often with involvement of students. District, regional, tertiary/academic and specialist psychiatric hospitals further all offer inpatient facilities (very limited in district hospitals, and only short term), at various length and intensity according to clinical profile. Many South African mental health professionals have long been recognising the importance of care transcending hospital settings, and have translated that into specialist outreach teams, where teams made up of psychiatrists and psychologists would visit key PHC clinics in the province at regular intervals, where people accessing outpatient care can renew their six-month medication scripts and possibly receive referrals to further care if required. There are several varied examples of this model of care. This includes pioneering work led by Carlo Gagiano in the Free State province in the 1980s and 1990s (Fourie & Gagiano 1988); outreach activities in Gauteng consisting of medical registrars operating under the guidance of senior psychiatrists (Robertson & Szabo 2017); and Assertive Community Intervention Teams (ACITs) – interdisciplinary teams that are made up of a medical officer, social worker, three psychiatric nurses and a psychiatrist – operating in the Western Cape (Botha et al. 2014).

The options for people suffering from chronic, severe and debilitating psychiatric conditions that require advanced levels of care, are limited. This limitation is extended to its extreme when the person in question does not have the funds to access private for-profit care. Essentially, this particular population are either cared for by their families (in many cases placing an extreme burden on an already overstretched household); placed in long-term care facilities operated by CSOs; or spends long stretches of time in state psychiatric facilities. Specialised psychiatric facilities remain the main provider of public mental health beds for inpatient care (Lund et al. 2012).

The services described thus far largely operate within the ambit of the state, but health services are also provided by a private sector, operating with the primary motivation of profit. This includes general or family practitioners, who are often a first point of call for mental disorder symptoms. The bulk of South Africa's mental health professionals – psychiatrists, psychologists and counsellors – work in private, independent offices, largely in urban areas. They often also contract their services out to a variety of private, for-profit hospitals, that include general hospitals, psychiatric and substance abuse rehabilitation facilities, and various step-down and day clinics. These service providers have had a contentious relationship with the state, no doubt aggravated during recent years by the Department of Health's increasingly combative stance against the private sector in promoting the National Health Insurance (NHI) agenda. That being said, South African legislation and policy provides ample ground for collaboration between the state and private agencies, and public-private-partnerships such as Life Esidimeni, as well as smaller scale contracting work by general practitioners, will become a central (if contested) feature of NHI plans. Many medical specialists, including those providing mental health care, work in both state and private spaces (Ashmore 2013).

All services highlighted thus far fall under the stewardship of the Department of Health, and largely occur in facilities. Beyond this sphere however, there are a range of less biomedically-driven services that are critically neglected, and also forms a key site of political contestation. Loosely labelled in Figure 2.1 as "Community Care", this sphere of actors and activities include residential care, which can be provided by families or caretakers, or by various non-profit CSOs. This includes substance abuse rehabilitation facilities; halfway homes; old age homes; general residential homes (little exclusion criteria in terms of illness or disability); and specialised living homes (facilities offering care for specified groups, for instance adults living with mild and moderate schizophrenia). There is no standardised or regulated package of care adopted by any of these caretakers, and the quality and content of care varies wildly – some offer little more than basics like food and shelter, while others may offer a range of additional services. The services rendered largely depends on funding and support. Some receive support from universities in terms of students providing basic therapeutic care (especially occupational therapy and psychology), and some receive assistance from local businesses in the form of food and cash donations. Many also receive backing and support from voluntary, faith-based organisations, such as churches and voluntary community support groups. Services include, among others, counselling and support group therapy; assistance with grant management and other administrative issues; protective workshops, arts and crafts. Importantly, in this sphere of services, traditional healers and faith-based counsellors also operate, and are often a first point of call in more rural areas of the country. The non-profit, community-based dimensions of mental health care in South Africa is governed by several departments, mainly the Department of Health, Department of Social Development, and, to a lesser extent, Department of Labour and the South African Police Service. Although tasks related to all sectors are outlined in the MHPF, there is little evidence of inter-sectoral mental health care – a gap that only becomes apparent in times of crisis.

In this chapter, a broad, succinct overview was given of major mental health care developments in South Africa, with a focus on its post-apartheid period. The goal was to construct a map of service providers and sectors that provide a continuum of care to people suffering from severe mental and neurological conditions. A map that will enable an analysis of the political structure and relations between state, private for-profit and civil society mental health care providers, at the centre of which is a group of people rendered increasingly vulnerable by dynamics far beyond their control. In the next chapter, we start this analysis by focusing on a dimension of mental health care that, in the contexts of Global Mental Health and a renewed agenda for mental health care in South Africa, have been critically neglected in local scientific discourse. The importance of the positioning and activities of CSOs in relation to the state has been substantially elevated after the Life Esidimeni crisis, and requires closer examination.

Notes

1 For a detailed exploration of the Smith Mitchell and Co activities during apartheid, see Ure (2015).

2 South Africa has produced many other world-class scientists involved in the mental health system, though these particular projects and people were especially well-positioned within the broader Global Mental Health discourse, and research activities were almost always conducted in parallel with similar activities in other LMICs (particularly India, Nepal, Ethiopia, Zimbabwe, Uganda and Nigeria). Collaborative networks also extended to key "Northern" institutions, specifically King's College London and London School of Hygiene and Tropical Medicine.

3 Collaboration between state and non-state mental health services[1]

Introduction

Major global investment has been made in public mental health service improvement during the past decade, exemplified by the WHO Mental Health Action Plan; the Movement for Global Mental Health; an increase in research investment (highlighted in several dedicated series in prestigious journals); and the inclusion of mental health as a priority under Sustainable Development Goal 3.4 (Collins et al. 2011; Richard Horton 2007; Patel, Boyce, Collins, Saxena, & Horton 2011; Patel & Saxena 2014; G. Thornicroft & Patel 2014; Tomlinson et al. 2009). The South African mental health community took advantage of the global mental health movement (Patel et al. 2011) by producing a comprehensive national mental health policy in 2012. The Mental Health Policy Framework and Strategic Plan 2013–2020 (MHPF) (National Department of Health 2013) is a comprehensive and ambitious document, focusing in broad strokes on improving mental health service delivery on primary, secondary and tertiary levels of the public health system. In step with post-apartheid legislation and health policy approaches, it re-affirms the responsibility of the state to provide public mental health services (section 8). Important steps have recently been taken towards integrating mental health care into the primary health care (PHC) system through a task-shifting approach (Jack et al. 2014; Lund, Tomlinson, & Patel 2016; Petersen & Lund 2011; Petersen, Lund, Bhana, & Flisher 2012; Petersen et al. 2017b). While various forms and types of integration have been conceptualised (Kodner 2009; Kodner & Spreeuwenberg 2002), integration is essentially a social process involving the management and delivery of a continuum of curative and preventative, multi-level health services, according to the needs of clients (World Health Organization 2008).

In South Africa, there is perhaps no more striking example of the consequences of the disintegration of mental health services than the Life Esidimeni tragedy. In this botched deinstitutionalisation attempt, the Gauteng Department of Health ended a long-standing public-private partnership with a major private hospital group, transferring 1 371 mental health service users from specialist care settings to CSOs during 2016 (Makgoba 2017). To date, more than 144 have died due to gross negligence, while an unknown number remains missing. The state purportedly followed global narratives that underline the primacy of deinstitutionalisation, despite a well-established historical account of the pitfalls of such strategies (Koyanagi, Bazelon, & L 2007; Morrow, Dagg, & Pederson 2008; Shen & Snowden 2014; Sheth 2009; Thornicroft, Deb, & Henderson 2016). At the minimum, the Life Esidimeni tragedy is a spectacular failure of collaboration between state and non-state parties, and laid bare serious dysfunction of referral, regulation, and information systems, as well as pointing to a lack of stewardship on a grand scale (Makgoba 2017). The incident was further complicated by a structural disjuncture in governance between the Department of Health (DoH; who oversee health facilities and services) and the Department of Social Development (DoSD; who regulates the activities and services of CSOs), speaking to a degree of siloed working in mental health service provision. Additionally, the incident unfolded in contexts where the relationship between the state and CSOs are fraught with conflict. In South Africa, the establishment of the National Association of Welfare Organisations and Non-profit Organisations (NAWONGO) led to a lengthy court case against the state for improved access to funding (Court 2010). For Ferguson (Ferguson 2006), this is part of a transnational phenomenon in LMICs, and similar conflicts emerged in India in the wake of the 2010 introduction of the Foreign Contribution Regulation Act. Importantly, the MHPF is geared towards addressing these crucial concerns, particularly improved collaborative activities.

The MHPF built on a host of post-apartheid mental health reform strategies that have repeatedly stressed the importance of state and non-state collaboration (van Rensburg & Fourie 2016; van Rensburg, Rau, Fourie, & Bracke 2016). Non-state health service providers include both for and not for profit organisations (Wolvaardt et al. 2008). For-profit organisations include private hospitals, clinics, mental health professionals, and physicians. On the non-profit space of the spectrum, non-governmental organisations (NGOs) provide mental health services to recipients who cannot afford private care, and may include organisations in different local, national and international capacities, with different approaches. NGOs refer to "a broad spectrum of voluntary associations that are entirely or largely independent of state and that are not primarily motivated by commercial concerns" (Najam 2000), and in South Africa traditional healers are also counted among these service providers (Campbell-Hall et al. 2010; Sorsdahl et al. 2009). NGOs have gradually been recognised as an important resource to tap into and have become key collaborating actors in LMICs, exemplified by global initiatives such as mhNOW and #NGOs4mentalhealth call to action (Kleinman et al. 2016).

Collaboration here involves voluntary inter-organisational participation – with mutual adjustments – in arrangements that encompass the distribution of responsibilities and rewards among collaborators (Axelsson & Axelsson 2006; Hill & Lynn 2003), resulting in the provision of a multi-organisational service delivery network (May & Winter 2009). Conceptually, two distinct (but intersecting) features of collaboration can be distinguished, namely the degree of collaboration, and the contexts behind collaborative activity (Wanna, 2008). Collaboration is a core feature of organisational integration-the vertical and horizontal forms of health services networking and collaboration, both formal and informal (Durbin, Goering, Streiner, & Pink 2006; Kodner & Spreeuwenberg 2002). In South Africa's pluralistic health system, this involves, to a certain degree, collaborative ties between state and non-state service providers.

Recently, world health leaders including Jim Yong Kim, president of the World Bank Group, and Margaret Chan, Director-General of the WHO, called for a collaborative response to mental health care strengthening that stresses community-level, integrated mental health care (Kleinman et al. 2016). While the apparent global and local supportive policy environment should be applauded, many challenges remain. Importantly, evidence of health service requirements for mental health integration scale-up (Semrau et al. 2015) and the organisation, planning, infrastructure, and inter-sectoral linkages of referral systems (Rathod et al. 2017) are left wanting. There is an identified need to explore the types and interactions of state and non-state actors providing health services in LMICs (Cammett & MacLean 2011). Simply put, improved coordination and stakeholder involvement are crucial in translating mental health policies into tangible outcomes (Hanlon et al. 2017), and increasing collaboration is an essential step for "mental health to come out of the shadows" (Kleinman et al. 2016, p. 2274). To this end, the aim of this study was to provide understanding of the nature and extent of mental health service collaboration among state and non-state service providers in the Mangaung Metropolitan District in the Free State province of South Africa. The nature of collaborative activities here refers to the structure, type and dynamics of relationships, while the extent refers to the degree of collaboration.

Methods

Setting

The study was conducted in the Mangaung Metropolitan District, in the Free State Province, South Africa. With a population of 759 693, the district includes a city and several small towns and villages. The district includes areas that were designated Bantustans (territory set aside for black inhabitants) during apartheid, and socio-economic and health inequities remain. In 2016, a poverty headcount of 5% was estimated (a compound measurement of 11 indicators of health, education, living standards and economic activity, resulting in an indication of the proportion of households that are "multidimensional poor"). In 2015, 27.8% of households received government grants and subsidies (Statistics South Africa 2016).

Approach and design

The study draws from a mixed methods research approach. Nestled in a pragmatic research paradigm (real-world oriented, problem-centred, pluralist practices), mixed methods here refer to the collection and integration of both quantitative and qualitative data towards forming a more complete understanding of a research topic (Cresswell 2014). The study was informed by social network analysis (SNA), and heeding to suggestions that SNA should not be only used as a descriptive tool and that its combination with other approaches yield better explanation (Marshall & Staeheli 2015; Wölfer, Faber, & Hewstone 2015), the study employed semi-structured interviews as well. The data collection, analysis and integration of the two methodologies were conducted sequentially, while maintaining the same approximate weight in importance. The study design therefore can be described as an equal status, sequential mixed methods design, the quantitative phase (SNA) preceding the qualitative phase (Johnson & Onwuegbuzie 2004). SNA is an effective method with which to explore integrated care and other health system concerns (Blanchet & James 2012; Goodwin 2010), and has been shown to be a useful way to explore inter-organisational linkages among health-oriented organisations in LMIC settings (Ermien Van Pletzen, Zulliger, Moshabela, & Schneider 2013) and mental health care integration (Lorant, Nazroo, Nicaise, & Group 2017; Nicaise, Dubois, & Lorant 2014; Nicaise et al. 2013). The procedures were informed by the steps described by Blanchet and James (Blanchet & James 2012). Accordingly, the study sought to (i) describe the set of actors and members of the network; (ii) characterise the relationships between actors; and (iii) analyse network structures.

Instrument development

The structured interview schedule (SNA data collection instrument) was developed based on sections of an existing instrument investigating cooperative relationships among human service organisations (Bruynooghe, Verhaeghe, & Bracke 2008). Questions related to the research study were added, including descriptive questions about the organisations and the nature of mental health services and referrals offered. Semi-structured interviews with key participants were guided by a schedule informed by Purdy's (Purdy 2012) Framework for Assessing Power in Collaborative Governance Processes combined with probes related to state and non-state interactions, mental health system dynamics, and state stewardship.

Data gathering

To obtain network data, three steps were followed. First, a list of state health care facilities in Mangaung Metropolitan was obtained from the Free State Department of Health (FSDoH). This included 41 PHC facilities, three district hospitals, one regional hospital, and one specialist psychiatric hospital. From October to November 2015, the 46 facilities on the list were visited, and the social network instrument was administered face-to-face with health care professionals in charge of mental health care in their respective facilities. This step produced a list of state and non-state service providers with whom state facilities collaborated in mental health care. Second, the non-state providers identified in this step were visited and the social network instrument was administered by trained researchers face-to-face to the person in charge of mental health care in each organisation. Third, an additional list of NGOs providing mental health services was obtained from Families South Africa (a local NGO who kept records of available NGOs in the district), that was also visited in a similar manner as in other organisations. In total, 20 NGOs were identified. Ultimately, a total network of 66 mental health service collaboration partners, both state and non-state, was identified across the district.

Following an initial analysis of this network, clusters of state and non-state collaboration were identified, from which eleven participants were identified for semi-structured interviews. These key informants were asked to identify additional influential actors in mental health service provision not yet identified during the research, resulting in another nine participants identified. Ultimately, 20 semi-structured interviews were conducted, with durations spanning 40 to 80 minutes. All participants identified during these processes were contacted for appointments, and following informed consent procedures, semi-structured interviews were conducted in their offices. All participants were fluent in English, and all interviews were conducted accordingly in English.

Data management and analysis

SNA data was electronically captured and structured in Microsoft Excel (Microsoft 2010) and transferred to Gephi Graph Visualization and Manipulation software (version 0.9.1) (NetBeans 2016) for network analyses. Basic descriptive analysis was performed, producing indications of node (mental health service providers) and edge (relationships) numbers; network diameter (the shortest distance between the two most distant nodes in the network); average path length (the average number of steps along the shortest paths for all possible pairs of network nodes); density (proportion of the potential network connections that are actual connections); average degree (an average calculation of the number of edges connected to each node); clustering coefficient (the degree to which nodes tend to cluster together in the network); eigenvector values (measures of the relative influence of nodes in a network), and authority rankings (indications of the relative importance of nodes in a network). Gephi's No Overlap algorithm and centrality function were applied to produce an illustration of the network that affords nodes with more centrality a larger size. Filters were applied to isolate different types of collaborations. Approximations of the weight of interaction among state

Table 3.1 List of state/non-state mental health collaborations

State facility		*Non-state facility*	
Code	*Services provided in collaboration*	*Code*	*Service provided*
PHC A3	Out-patient drug treatment	NGO A2	Housing, rehab, treatment adherence
PHC A8	Out-patient drug treatment	NGO A1	Social/welfare services, psychotherapy
		NGO A2	Housing/rehab, treatment adherence
		NGO A4	Housing/rehab
		NGO A5	Substance abuse rehab and prevention
		NGO A7	Housing, treatment adherence
PHC A10	Out-patient drug treatment	NGO A1	Social/welfare services, psychotherapy
SH A1	Acute and serious case processing; social/ welfare services	NGO A1	Social/welfare services, psychotherapy
		NGO A4	Housing/rehab
PHC B12	Out-patient drug treatment	NGO B1	Housing, treatment adherence
DH B1	Out-patient drug treatment; acute and serious case processing	NGO B1	Housing, treatment adherence

(split into primary and hospital level) and non-state service providers were calculated in Excel.

The qualitative phase of the research focused on two groups of participants: 1) collaborating state and non-state collaborating service providers (Table 3.1), and 2) key informants (Table 3.2). Semi-structured interviews were audio recorded and transcribed verbatim to Microsoft Word (Microsoft 2010). Transcriptions were transferred to NVivo10 (QSR International 2016) for management during analysis. Interview transcripts were thematically analysed (Saldaña 2014). Pre-determined themes were deductively derived from the SNA instrument, namely, *Available mental health services*, *Reasons for collaboration*, and *Quality, effectiveness, efficiency of care*. *Power dynamics* emerged inductively during the data analysis process. Themes and their content were negotiated among three researchers to remove overlap or irrelevance from the data. Direct quotations – de-identified – are used to support thematic categorisation.

Ethical considerations

All research participants were informed of the purpose of the research and their role in it both verbally and in writing. Signed informed consent was obtained

Table 3.2 List of key informant positions and affiliations

Position	*Affiliation*
State	
Senior psychologist	Government department; Specialist hospital
Programme director	Government department
Psychiatrist	Psychiatry outreach team; District hospital
Psychologist	District hospital
Mental health nurse	District hospital
Mental health nurse	PHC clinic
Non-state	
Case worker	Non-profit organisation
CEO	Private for-profit psychiatric hospital
Director	Non-profit organisation

from participants, and data anonymity and confidentiality were achieved by assigning codes to data sources. Participants were offered freedom of participation, and none opted out of the study. Ethical clearance was obtained from the Stellenbosch University Research Ethics Committee: Human Research (Ref: HS1156/2015), and permission to conduct the research was obtained from the FSDoH.

Study findings

Extent of collaboration

As shown in Figure 3.1, a striking feature of the network of mental health service providers is the centrality of hospitals, especially the state psychiatric hospital (SH A1). Three distinct network groupings can be observed. The largest of the three is the city of Bloemfontein, which helps explain the larger concentration of service providers – especially NGOs. The two smaller groupings denote small towns which previously were situated in an apartheid-era Bantustan (Botshabelo and Thaba Nchu), resource-poor and geographically removed from specialist services.

Table 3.3 provides an overview of descriptive network statistics. The total network had 66 nodes (mental health service providers), and 175 edges (relationships in the network). The network diameter – the largest distance between two nodes – was six, meaning that it took six connections to join the two service providers farthest apart from each other in terms of collaborative relationships. The average length of the relationship paths between nodes was almost three (Table 3.3: Average path length = 2.9). The low number of indirect relationships is also reflected by an overall low level of network density (Table 3.3: Density = 0.041), as well as by a low average degree (Table 3.3: Average Degree = 2.652). The clustering coefficient – a calculation

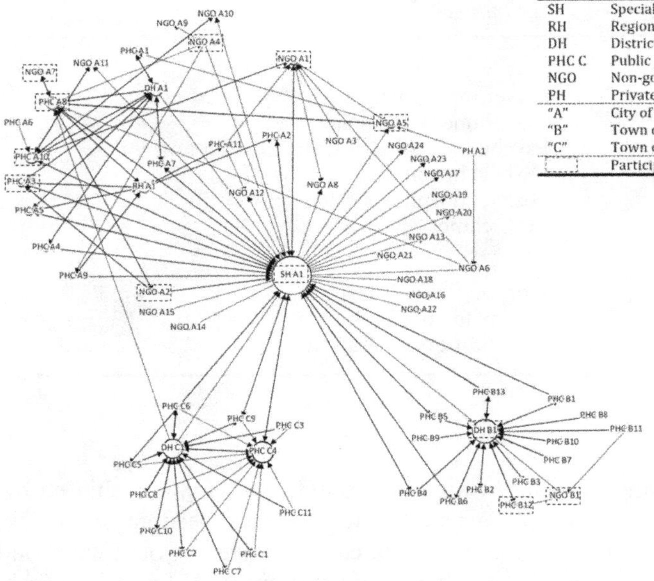

Legend	
SH	Specialist public hospital
RH	Regional public hospital
DH	District public hospital
PHC C	Public primary health care clinic
NGO	Non-governmental organisation
PH	Private hospital
"A"	City of Bloemfontein
"B"	Town of Botshabelo
"C"	Town of Thaba Nchu
[dashed box]	Participants selected for interviews

Figure 3.1 Total network.

of the probability that two separate nodes connected to a given node are connected two, therefore indicating clusters of triangular connections among nodes – was also relatively low at 0.247. Estimated between zero and one, this suggests few clusters of collaborative relationships throughout the network. It is important to note that the statistical averages presented here conceal a substantial discrepancy in terms of a high number of edges attached to selected service providers while other service providers have only a few edges attached to it. This reflects considerable inequality in the network, along with suggesting a hierarchical structure characterised by a broad base and a narrow top. The state-run psychiatric hospital (SH A1) was the most powerful node in the network. Apart from its superior degree centrality, it was the most influential service provider according to its high eigenvector centrality value (1.0) and its high network authority (0.385) relative to other nodes.

Proportional interactions – that is, the proportion of the total possible interactions between groups, indicated by a number between 0 and 1 – among different service providers were analysed in three groups: hospitals, PHC facilities (both state-driven), and NGOs. Given the disparity in distribution of mental health professionals between primary care on the one hand, and secondary and specialist care on the other, state facilities were divided accordingly. As shown in Figure 3.1, most interactions took place between hospitals and PHC clinics, with comparatively less interactions between these two

Table 3.3 Descriptive network statistics

Nodes	*Edges*	*Diameter*	*Ave. path length*	*Density*	*Ave. degree*	*Ave clustering coefficient*	*Highest eigenvector value*	*Highest authority*
66	175	6	2.90	0.041	2.652	0.247	SH A1: 1.0	SH A1: 0.385

Nodes	66
Edges	175
Diameter	6
Ave. path length	2.90
Density	0.041
Ave. degree	2.652
Ave clustering coefficient	0.247
Highest eigenvector value	SH A1: 1.0
Highest authority	SH A1: 0.385

groups and non-state facilities. The highest number of relationships between state and non-state was the referral of patients from hospitals to non-state facilities. A possible reason here – described in the qualitative section – is the concentration of state mental health professionals in hospital care, who might be more likely to collaborate with non-state actors.

Nature of state and non-state mental health service collaboration

Range of services offered

The semi-structured interviews shed light on the range and nature of the core services that were offered by different service providers in the district. State and non-state service providers seemingly provided different kinds of care to mental health service users. The hierarchical structure of state health facilities according to primary, secondary and tertiary levels were concomitant with concentration and availability of specialist human resources for health. The specialist psychiatric hospital provided a broad range of services across all ages – outpatient drug therapy, in-patient services (that included occupational therapy), psychotherapy, treatment adherence, alcohol and drug rehabilitation, and forensic and social services. The hospital's ties to the university provided a pool (albeit a relatively small one) of specialists, especially psychiatrists, clinical psychologists, social workers, psychiatric nurses, and occupational therapists. As the SNA results suggested, there seemed to be a geographical inequality in terms of distribution of types of services, the more socially-aligned services were more concentrated in more urbanised areas (Figure 3.2). In more rural areas, participants mentioned that some mental health service users access care from traditional healers, though no formal referral or collaboration was found between the participants and possible traditional healers in the district.

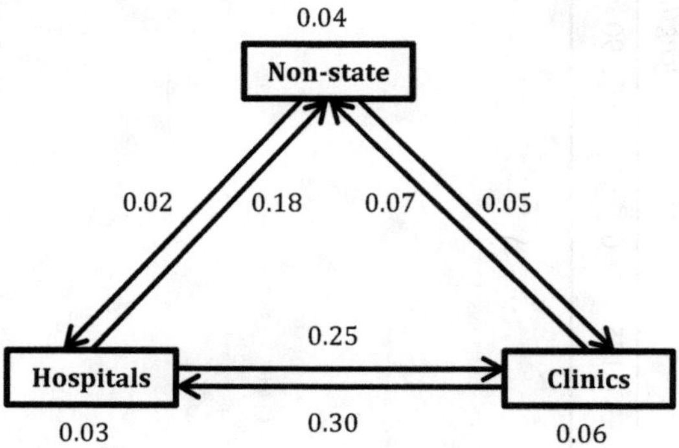

Figure 3.2 Proportional interactions between service providers.

Some of the NGOs provided a range of basic care services, of which housing was especially prolific. Mental health service users were brought there by their families, and the NGOs took care of them – usually in a restructured private home, with several beds and mattresses for mental health service users. Instances were found where as many as 30 mental health service users (both male and female) were housed in a three-bedroom house, with one bathroom. Nevertheless, their core services included housing, food, and treatment adherence. Mental health service users based in places like this did seemingly not have access to any psychotherapy or rehabilitation, and their care comprised of drug adherence and basic human needs. A key service that emerged during this narrative is the "containment and management" of mental health service users. This is illustrated below:

> *Yes, they escape. All of them, they will pop the windows. They break the windows. At night. We do not sleep then. We walk around, check the place.*
> (CC_NGO1)

Very little psychotherapy, rehabilitation and support existed outside large public hospitals in urban areas. This was apart from fee for service facilities, which had little contact with public health services due to their for-profit motive. An especially strong actor in this sense was a local NGO who specialised in assisting mental health service users who are not able to afford private mental health care, employing social workers. Their core service package included home-based psychotherapy, group therapy, social support, community awareness and education campaigns, and referrals to other necessary services. Some NGOs did not specialise in mental health care, and rather encompassed it as part of its main focus. Examples include an organisation that provided support and services in line with anti-occultism, alcohol and drug rehabilitation facilities, and organisations focusing on geriatric care. Geriatric facilities were cited as a way in which care can be extended to mental health service users, given the presence of medical and around the clock care. One faith-based organisation provided a spectrum of services, as explained here:

> *We have seven main services. The old age centre, family care, child and youth care, adoption services that are international and national, and then also hospital care and disability care. Then we also have substance dependence programmes, the prevention and alleviation of poverty, and forensic services.*
> (CC_NGO4)

The only for-profit organisation identified in the network was a private psychiatric hospital, with significant human resource capital, but very little collaboration with other service providers. Their package of care was extensive, and included psychotherapy, dietary care, physiotherapy, and frequent access to psychologists and psychiatrists. This particular facility was established following the exchange of psychiatric beds in private hospitals for more profitable surgical beds. Given a perceived rise in mental health needs (especially among middle-class populations who have medical insurance), this market gap was filled. Many of the mental health professionals employed by the facility have dual roles, occupying positions in both the private hospital as well as providing services in state hospitals. The profit motive of this particular facility restricted collaboration with NGOs and state facilities. The little service exchange that did occur unfolded in cases where mental medical aid funds were depleted, viewed with disdain by some participants:

> *The only time that we engage with them is when the money runs out and then they send them to us, so that actually happens a lot. Yes, around June, July, the patients come from private and then their funds are depleted.*
>
> (SW_TH)

Referrals

SNA findings suggested that PHC facilities tended to refer mental health service users with perceived serious mental conditions, as well as acute cases that often involved psychosis, to hospitals. Hospitals tended to refer discharged mental health service users to PHC facilities for outpatient drug treatment. An important point of collaboration between state and non-state service providers was referral of mental health service users to NGOs that provided housing, basic needs and treatment adherence. Specialised services such as drug and alcohol rehabilitation and psychosocial therapy and rehabilitation were only concentrated in a few NGOs. Available family support services were sparse (Table 3.4).

Findings from the semi-structured interviews suggested that public health facilities tended to follow provincial referral policy. In this vein, PHC clinics generally screened mental health service users for signs and symptoms of mental illness, and referred them accordingly. In serious cases, mental health

Table 3.4 Types of network interactions

Reason for collaboration	*Number of interactions*	
	n	%
Outpatient drug therapy	*58*	33.14
Acute cases	*42*	24.0
Serious cases	*34*	19.43
Housing	*25*	14.29
Drug and alcohol rehab	*6*	3.43
Psycho-therapy	*6*	3.43
Family support	*4*	2.28

service users were referred upwards to district hospitals, which referred upwards to the regional hospital in the district, which in turn referred to the psychiatric hospital. Hospitals in turn referred mental health service users downwards to PHC clinics for outpatient treatment. Given the paucity of mental health expertise in PHC clinics, an outreach team made up of medical residents in psychiatry and clinical psychologists visited certain clinics in the district in order to increase access to treatment initiation and adaption. Mental health service users are booked for a predetermined date and then seen by the outreach team at a clinic or hospital. Cases deemed to be serious were referred to district hospitals where mental health service users were assessed for a period of 72 hours before being referred further (as stipulated in the Mental Health Care Act). This was perceived to be a necessary policy to prevent the overburdening of the specialist psychiatric hospital: "We do not want to be flooded and stuff" (CP_TH).

However, the capacity of district hospitals to offer this particular service was questioned, particularly in terms of adequate space and available mental health professionals. Apart from the official provincial referral system, which dictates that public health facilities have to refer mental health service users to other public health facilities according to a pre-determined referral list, very few state facilities had any formal referral rules in place for referral to non-state service providers. In this vein, the social work unit at the psychiatric hospital was the exception, being a key point of collaboration with NGOs.

Reasons for mental health service collaboration

In the second phase of the network analysis, filters were used to isolate relationships that were identified by the research participants. During the semi-structured interviews, participants were asked to name the main mental health service that they provide in relation to other mental health service providers. These parts of the service delivery network are presented in Figures 3.3–3.9, and in Table 3.4. Seven different reasons for collaborative relationships among service providers were identified by participants: Outpatient pharmaceutical care; Serious cases; Drug and alcohol rehabilitation; Psychotherapy and psychosocial rehabilitation; Acute cases; Family support; and Housing and treatment adherence It should be noted that these relationships are not clear-cut, and that many overlaps occur. From the network depictions there is a suggestion of network density disparity between biomedically-oriented services (Outpatient drug therapy, Acute cases, Serious cases) and social support and psychotherapeutically-oriented services (Housing and treatment adherence, Drug and alcohol rehabilitation, Psychotherapy and psychosocial rehabilitation, and Family support). That is, the continuum of mental health care seems to be more skewed towards biomedical than psychosocial approaches. This schism is further bolstered by disparities in terms of the balance of biomedical services subsisting predominantly in the state sphere, while psychosocial services were largely rooted in the sphere of non-state

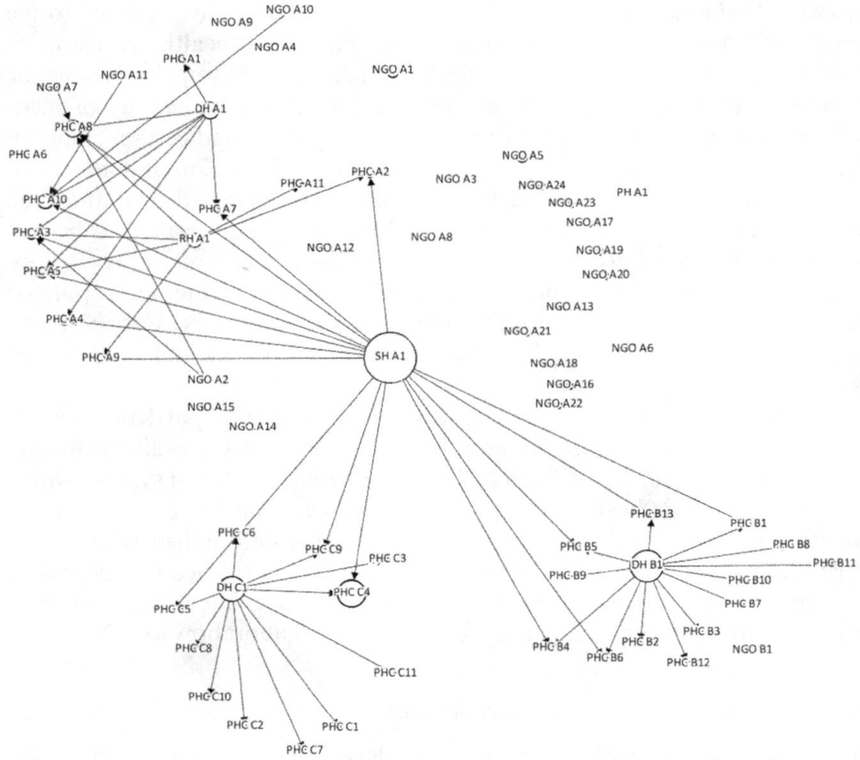

Figure 3.3 Outpatient pharmaceutical care.

services (see Table 3.4 for a breakdown of number of interactions per service). The apparent biomedical-psychosocial disjuncture was also underlined in terms of a sector split between the DoH and the DoSD. DoH is the steward of health, and in charge of health facilities. DoSD leads psychosocial rehabilitation and housing, while also regulating the NGO sector. The suggestion therefore is that not only is a disparity between state and non-state services, but also between the DoH and DoSD.

Semi-structured interviews further illuminated the reasons for collaboration. The point was made – especially by PHC clinics – that in the absence of adequate community-based assistance for mental health service users, there is a great deal of state reliance on NGOs. NGOs created a link between the state health system and mental health service users in the surrounding communities. By identifying people in need, and providing them with housing and basic needs, these organisations also linked them up with their local PHC clinics and district hospitals for psychiatric care. Facilities with a presence of social

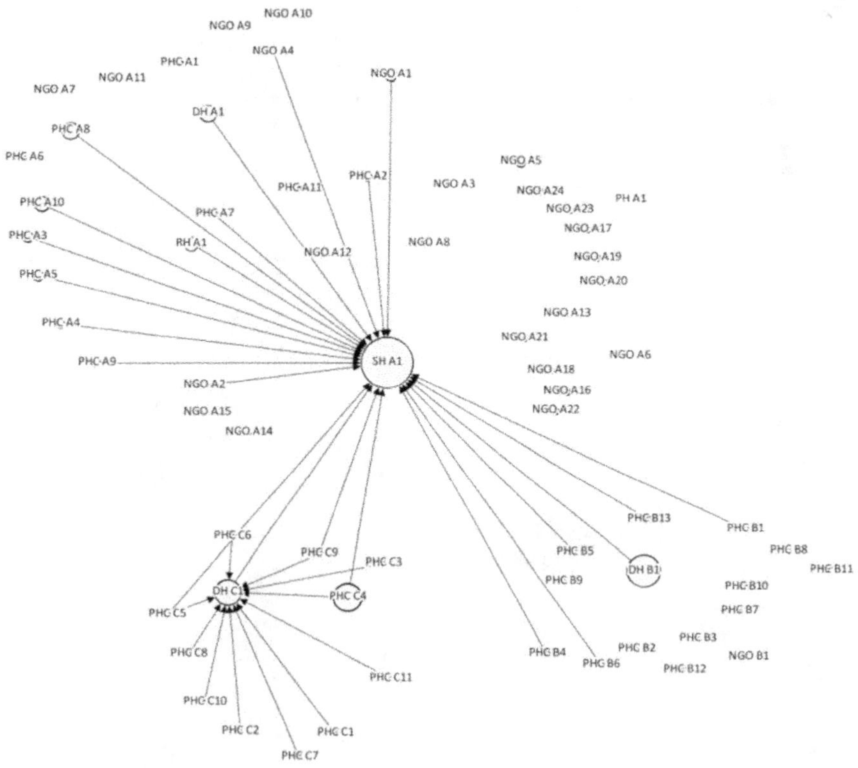

Figure 3.4 Serious cases.

work as a core service voiced appreciation for collaboration with NGOs. This said, singular participants viewed NGOs providing mental health services with contempt and suspicion, and did not see a necessity to collaborate. Such participants were of the opinion that the state should solely be responsible for service provision, and recommended that collaboration with NGOs that provide housing services should be replaced with state institutionalisation of mental health service users. The most important reasons for collaboration between state and non-state service providers were drug and alcohol rehabilitation; psychotherapy and psychosocial rehabilitation; family support; and housing and treatment adherence. While all these functions fall in the regulatory sphere of the DoSD, there was some overlap with the DoH in that state health facilities referred mental health service users to NGOs that provide housing and treatment adherence. It was not entirely clear to what extent such NGOs were regulated. Several state health care workers voiced concern about the conditions of these NGOs, but very few had visited these facilities, citing NGOs as the purview of the DoSD and social workers. NGOs in turn

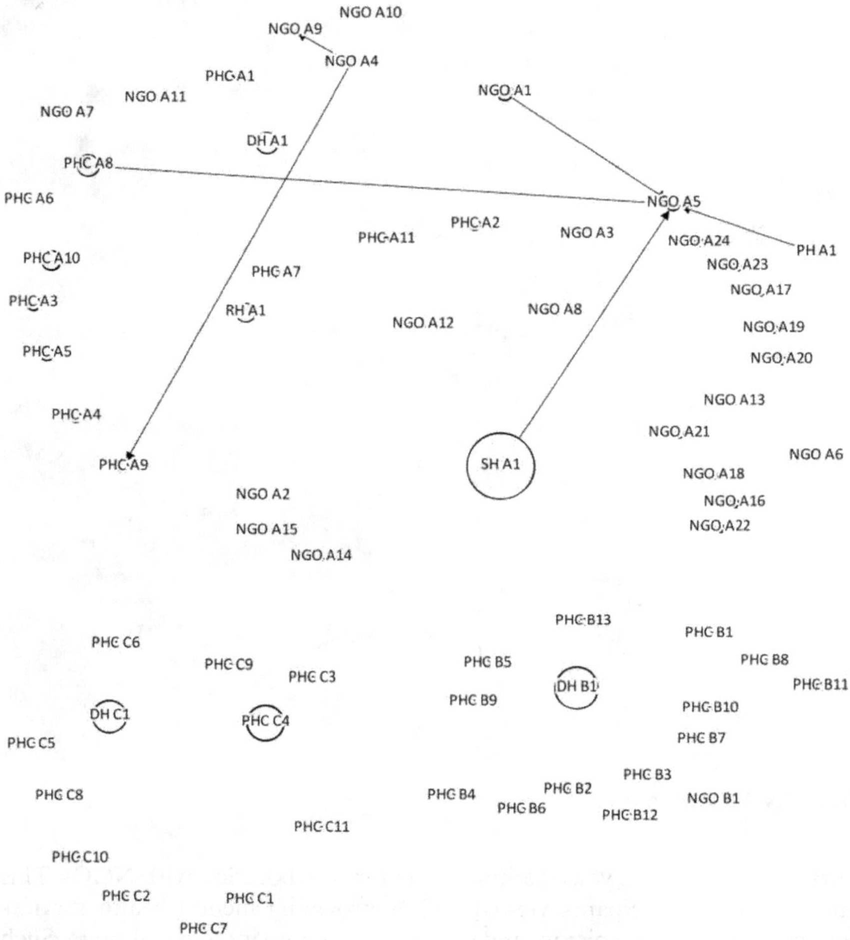

Figure 3.5 Drug and alcohol rehab.

relied heavily on state health care facilities for the clinical and pharmaceutical treatment of their clients, even though some alleged that mental health service users are neglected when seeking care in state facilities. The state psychiatric facility collaborated with NGOs in terms of the processing of statutory and forensic cases, as well as relying on non-state social workers to access communities to follow up on deinstitutionalised mental health service users. In cases where mental health service users became violent or experienced psychosis, the local police station was contacted for transport support. Many participants mentioned difficulties in transporting mental health service users suffering from psychosis between facilities. Subjectivities of dangerousness and risk

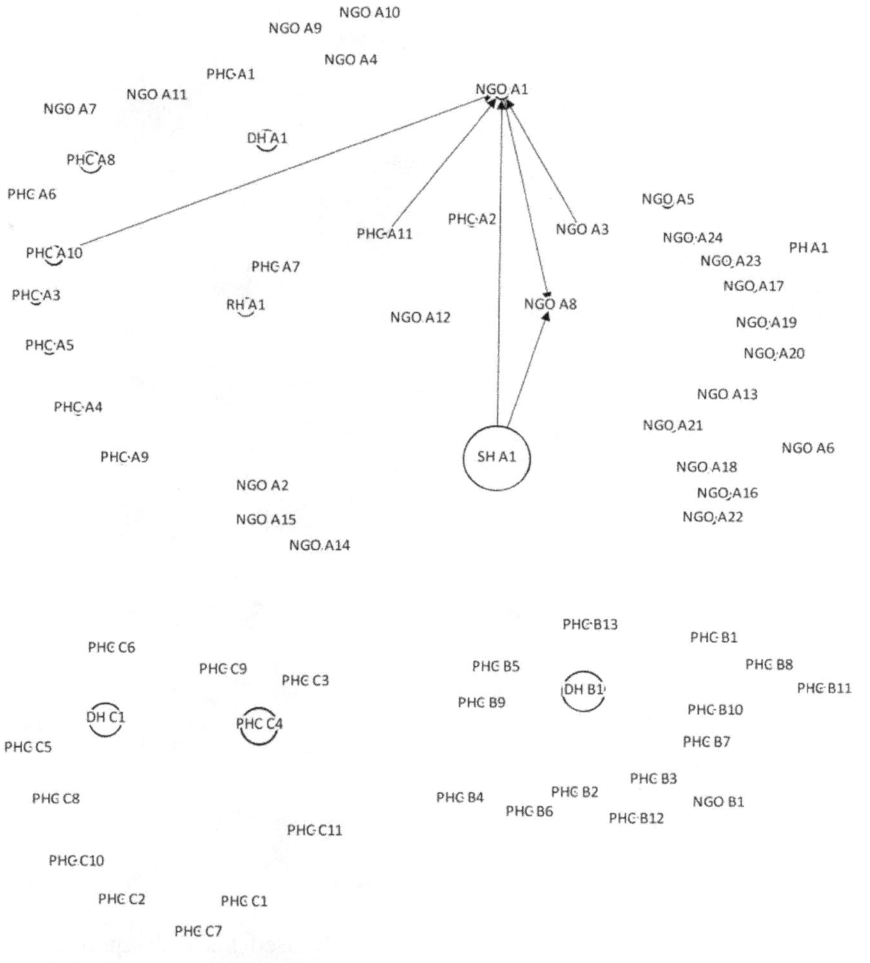

Figure 3.6 Therapy and rehab.

emerged, that were tied together with inflections of stigmatising attitudes of state health care workers towards mental illness. A general unwillingness of state health facilities to "deal" with mental health service users who exhibited psychotic episodes was described, and ambulance services were dismissed as a possible transportation option. Despite an apparent lack of training and willingness of police officers to assist, transporting mental health service users was seen as a police function, because "… we can't carry the patient of something into a car. It's not as if he will say, 'please, thank you I will get in', and drive away" (CC_NGO8). In the absence of police assistance and ambulance service availability, local NGOs were asked to assist with transportation. One

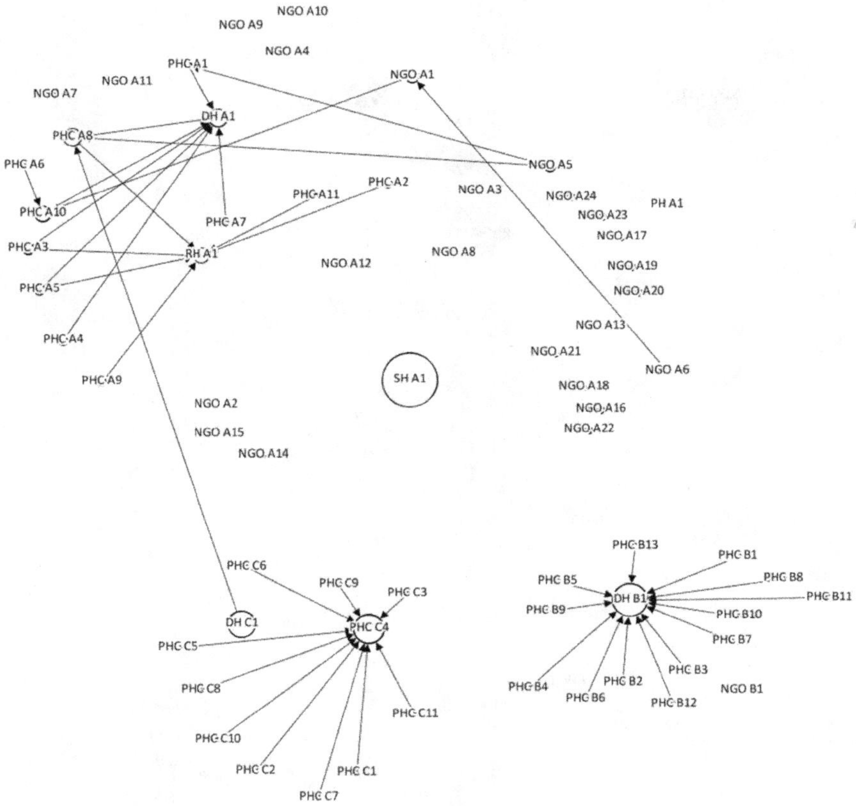

Figure 3.7 Acute cases.

NGO participant mentioned that he frequently used his pick-up truck to move mental health service users from state health facilities to his housing facilities, stating that "They want to get rid of that person. They then they phone us" (CC_NGO3).

Power dynamics

Power emerged in several forms. As suggested by the SNA results, state hierarchy alongside provincial health service referral policy was a particularly strong primer for collaboration. Power in terms of network centrality (Figure 3.1) was closely associated with professional capacity. Accordingly, hospitals with stronger concentrations of mental health professionals seemingly received and referred more mental health service users, resulting in a hospital-centric referral system. One participant expressed frustration

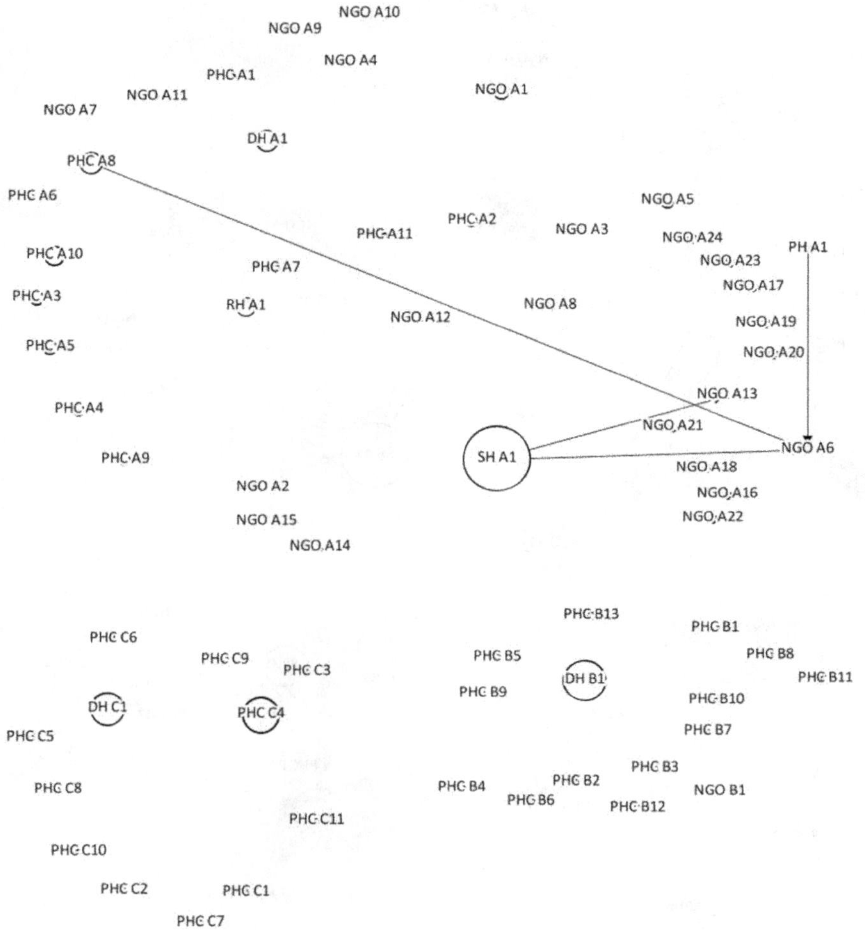

Figure 3.8 Family support.

that – despite regular awareness – PHC level state-run facilities did not refer mental health service users to them for further care and support, rather opting for hospital referrals:

> *It is a farce, because this organisation is 68 years old and they don't even know our name.*
>
> (CC_NGO2)

This observation and the salience of professional power was supported by a state mental health nurse, who expressed unwillingness to refer mental

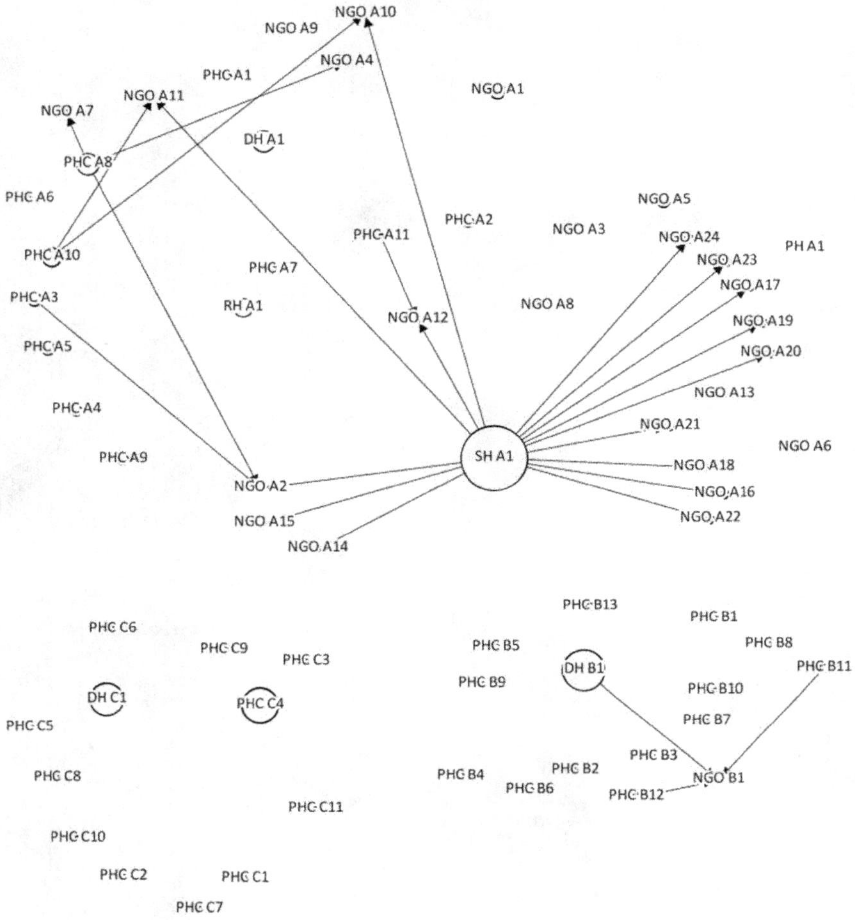

Figure 3.9 Housing and treatment adherence.

health service users to non-state actors due to a perceived lack of psychiatric expertise on their part:

> *We advise them to not go there…Because I don't think they are with us. You can see other referrals. They are not with us. There's no private doctor who can think he can manage psychiatry.*
>
> (PN_DH2)

It emerged that different mental health professionals equated different sources of power. A clinical psychologist remarked that nobody had a voice in mental health care, except for psychiatrists. Psychiatry and clinical psychology was almost exclusively concentrated in hospitals, and PHC clinics relied heavily on the psychiatric outreach team to process mental health service users' clinical treatment regimes. This source of power was also evident in terms of NGOs linking up with state hospitals (and not with PHC clinics). The significance of this power dynamic was particularly reflected in the reluctance of some participants to refer mental health service users to facilities outside the state services sphere – supporting the suggestion of weak state and non-state service providers (Figure 3.2). The biomedical slant and clinical nature of state facilities – compounded by the apparent chasm between the DoH and DoSD – further blocked participants from more holistic approaches that take into account living conditions and employment as key elements of mental health care. In this vein, a crucial form of professional power in facilitating state and non-state collaboration was the influence of social work as a profession. There seemed to be a suggestion that social workers are key agents in bridging the state and non-state collaboration gap, and several instances emerged that substantiate this deduction. For example, state social workers had power to provide forensic and specialised treatment for mental health service users, while non-state social workers had access to community settings and people's homes. These services were an important point of collaboration between the state psychiatric hospital and an NGO.

Quality, effectiveness and efficiency of care

Finally, when probed on what is necessary to improve mental health services, study participants made several recommendations. Efficient health information and referral systems were viewed to be dysfunctional, making tracking mental health service user care almost impossible – especially between state and non-state service providers. This is illustrated in the following outtake:

> *You're giving a date and say: "Go there". So as soon as this person walks out of here, we don't know. Because they never bring back, like even our patients themselves never bring it back to us and say: "I went there and this is what happened". So we're not sure what happens at the end.*
>
> (PN_PHCC3)

The need for reliable and appropriate transportation for moving mental health service users between service providers was widely discussed. This need was especially pressing in cases where there was reliance on police assistance with transporting people experiencing psychotic episodes to hospitals. District hospitals – who are supposed to admit and evaluate people suffering from psychosis for a mandated 72-hour period – lack both the appropriate infrastructure and mental health professionals to achieve this objective, often leading to mental health service users being discharged before receiving adequate care. Drug stock-outs were mentioned by some participants on PHC level. NGOs providing housing and treatment support highlighted a need for state funding, better physical infrastructure and facilities, and more clinical support from state mental health professionals. Shortages of mental health professionals, especially in community and in rural settings, were highlighted. A lack of state stewardship, leadership and governance in mental health care was discussed by both state and non-state participants, both on provincial and national levels. As mentioned above, and related to this challenge, NGOs called for alternative funding structures, as well as for improved compensation for services rendered. Financial need was discussed by the bulk of participants, which relate to operational costs, infrastructure, and human resources – all translating into the quality of care provided. This was simply illustrated as follows:

> *Without money, we cannot provide services. You can't fill your car with petrol and you can't drive to see your clients. I can't drive to conduct my group sessions and drive to go do community work.*
>
> (CC_NGO2)

Discussions

Despite global mental health service improvements during the past decade (Collins et al. 2011; Richard Horton 2007; Patel et al. 2011; Patel & Saxena 2014; G. Thornicroft & Patel 2014; Tomlinson et al. 2009), and the introduction of a dedicated mental health care policy in South Africa (National Department of Health 2013), our findings suggest that much is left to be achieved at local levels of service delivery. The MHPF adds to calls underlining the primacy of strong collaboration between state and non-state service providers (Janse van Rensburg & Fourie 2016; Millward, Provan, Fish, Isett, & Huang 2009; Savage, Taylor, Rotarius, & Buesseler 1997), though it may seem that the 'wicked problem' of mental health in health policy (Hannigan & Coffey 2011) indeed produces few success stories (Mur-Veeman, Van Raak, & Paulus 1999).

Regarding the extent of state and non-state mental health service collaboration, the network data suggested a sparse, relatively weakly integrated network with low network density and average degree. Worryingly, and in contrast to policy directives – centrality measures suggested that the collaboration network was largely dominated by hospitals, particularly by the state psychiatric hospital. The absence of contact between service providers and traditional healers was surprising. This support previous qualitative findings from South Africa that suggested a lack of collaboration between the formal health sector and traditional healers in mental health, compared to programmes such as HIV (Campbell-Hall et al. 2010). Indications that a large proportion of South Africans seek mental health care from traditional healers (Sorsdahl et al. 2009) elevate the importance of this collaborative gap. Ultimately, this particular network was weakly integrated in terms of sub-optimal primary and community care and the domination of acute care sectors (Mur-Veeman, van Raak, & Paulus 2008). The complete absence of formal service agreements further puts the network at the weak end of the integration spectrum (Nicaise et al. 2013). The necessity of NGOs as conduits to communities becomes pressing in spaces where the formal state is relatively weak (Donahue 2004), and our study add to previous indications that very little mental health service collaboration occurs on district-level in South Africa (Hanlon et al. 2014).

There is a distinct silence in academic literature on mental health service networks in LMICs. In one of very few empirical articles related to the subject, Van Pletzen and colleagues (Ermien Van Pletzen et al. 2013) explored partnership networks of health-related NGOs in South Africa, finding wide variations in numbers, resources, and orientation of partnership networks. Studies that focus on state and non-state sector collaboration remain crucially under-researched. This is an important omission, given the development potential of social network analysis to foster stronger state and non-state collaboration (Provan et al. 2005). In South Africa, this ideal is crucial in the wake of the Life Esidimeni tragedy. The country's substantial disease burden, as well as its significant inequalities and inequities in terms of race, sex, spatiality and access to health care – a result of centuries of colonialism and apartheid rule – further elevates the need for improved service integration (Coovadia et al. 2009b; Fourie, 2006; Harris et al. 2011; Harrison 2009c; Bongani M Mayosi et al. 2012; H. Van Rensburg & Engelbrecht 2012a). Our findings underline the persisting legacy of apartheid policy, in that rural, poorly resourced areas still suffer from a lack of service access. This is not to say that quality services are readily available in urban areas, and inequitable access in terms of richly resourced private for-profit and less well-endowed public service remains a crucial structural challenge in mental health service reform. By drawing from the diverse group of service providers on district level and therefore pooling resources, much progress can be made towards universal coverage (Axelsson & Axelsson 2006).

Similar to other contexts (M.-J. Fleury, Grenier, Bamvita, Wallot, & Michel 2012; Mur-Veeman, Hardy, Steenbergen, & Wistow 2003; Nicaise et al. 2014), several different points of collaboration – though limited – emerged. Non-state service providers largely relied on state facilities for outpatient pharmaceutical care; serious psychiatric cases; drug and alcohol rehabilitation; and psychotherapy and psychosocial rehabilitation. State facilities in turn relied on non-state sectors for drug and alcohol rehabilitation; psychotherapy and psychosocial rehabilitation; family support; and housing and treatment adherence. Following the Life Esidimeni tragedy, housing and treatment adherence was an especially salient point of collaboration. Instances of distrust in the capacities of NGOs to provide this service, as well as concern over the conditions of some of these NGOs and lack of regulatory oversight, were not entirely unfounded. While investigating the conditions of NGOs falls beyond the scope of this study, the fissures between the DoH and DoSD spheres of governance help to explain some of the main features of the Life Esidimeni tragedy: a breakdown in coordination and communication between state departments and NGOs, lack of regulatory oversight, and importantly, poor stewardship. It is telling that the DoSD does not feature in the official report into the tragedy, despite being stewards of the NGO sector (Makgoba 2017).

Indeed, the nature of collaboration between state and non-state mental health service providers was characterised by an apparent fragmentation between the governance spheres of the DoH and the DoSD, in other words, between medicine and the social. There was an apparent schism between medical-oriented services (outpatient drug therapy, acute cases, serious cases), provided mostly by the state, and socially oriented services (housing and treatment adherence, drug and alcohol rehabilitation, psycho-therapy, family support), provided largely by non-state services providers. This is not a challenge unique to South Africa, and a lack of health and social service integration within delivery networks has also been noted in high-income countries such as Belgium, the Netherlands, England, and Canada (Fleury et al. 2012; Mur-Veeman et al. 2003; Nicaise et al. 2014). Similar bodies of evidence from LMICs are unfortunately almost non-existent. Knocking down the "Berlin Wall" between health and social care has been an onerous and persistent challenge faced by governments globally (Dickinson & Glasby 2010), and its presence in the present case was telling. The primary goal of state and non-state collaboration is to produce outcomes that cannot be achieved by separate actors and sectors (Dickinson & Glasby 2010). The inter and intra fragmentation of coordination between government (DoH, DoSD, and police) and NGOs can result in mental health service users not receiving the most basic elements of care such as safe transport and shelter, as was vividly illustrated in the Life Esidimeni case. To a large degree, fragmented mental health care on organisational level boils down to failures in stewardship and leadership. Participation in a mental health service network is closely tied to effective leadership, determined by leaders whose interpretations and motivations influence the choice of collaborative partners (Purdy 2012). The responsibility for fostering multisectoral and state and non-state collaboration is at the feet of provincial government (South African Government 2004), who need to fulfil their constitutional mandate. The critical mechanisms of mental health stewardship and leadership in this network is described elsewhere, with particular attention paid to the promise of regular stakeholder roundtable discussions as a governance strategy with which to foster stronger collaboration (Janse van Rensburg et al. 2018).

Many challenges to organisational integration are rooted in relations among network members, each whom have their own interests and agency (Provan et al. 2005). In many instances, collaboration serves ulterior political motives, taking on a "perfunctory, cosmetic" veneer (Wanna 2008)10. Our findings revealed power dynamics – a key feature of integrated health care policy implementation (Erasmus & Gilson 2008; Gilson & Raphaely 2008; Janse van Rensburg et al. 2016; Lehmann & Gilson 2015) – in different forms. State government hierarchy and provincial health system referral policy were seemingly strong influences in collaboration. Authoritative power – "power over" – is firmly couched in the hierarchical health service organisation of South African districts (Lehmann & Gilson 2013). Implementation of integrated care policy is difficult in divergent networks with significant power disparities and conflicting perceptions of service delivery (Fleury, Mercier, & Denis 2002). Resistance to such power structures can be found in health care workers bypassing traditional lines of authority, as well as in coalitions between NGOs, as has been the case in the establishment of NAWONGO (Janse van Rensburg 2018). These features of power require further unpacking, similar to other work on power and resistance in health service provision (Lehmann & Gilson 2013 2015; Scott et al. 2014).

Limitations

The cross-sectional study design may have limited the possibility of valid claims – network depictions require frequent revision given the longitudinal dynamics of inter-organisational service collaboration (Mur-Veeman et al. 2003). The strategy followed to identify the mental health network in this study has an inherent drawback, in that isolated mental health service providers are under-represented. It could be that the identified network is not all-inclusive, since some organisations that provide mental health services might just not be effectively linked to the network under scrutiny. Genuine mental health service reform requires sincere participation of all stakeholders (Fleury, Mercier, & Denis 2002), and both organisational and population perspectives inform integrated mental health service networks (Fleury 2005). Our study did not include the voices of mental health service users and their families, which certainly opens avenues for further research. Referral rates are a common indicator of inter-organisational collaboration (Craven & Bland 2006). The weight of network referral linkages – an original goal of the study – could not be determined due to the almost non-existence of coordinated, valid monitoring data. An important facet of fostering integrated mental health services lies in the measurement of system performance by means of indicators that transcends policy domains (Plagerson 2015), a feature sorely missing from the present district health information system.

Recommendations

The Life Esidimeni crisis (Makgoba 2017) in many ways exemplified South Africa's protracted struggle towards comprehensive public mental health care provisioning. LMIC mental health services have been typified by resource investment in the clinical, facility-based aspects of mental health care with a focus on symptomatic and short-term care (Saraceno & Dua 2009). The social dimensions of care have been shifted to the sphere of NGOs, who are often inadequately supported, disparate and not well integrated with state health services, rendering the continuum of care disjointed (Inge Petersen, Lund, & Stein 2011). A re-assessment of funding models is required here, as investments need to follow mental health service users from hospitals and clinics to the community. Crucially, integrated health services require inter-institutional arrangements such as policy and financial re-structuring, but also attitudinal, cultural and power changes and professionals' consensus on the division of labour (Mur-Veeman et al. 2003). In order to create and foster appropriate models of integrated community-based care, an expansion is required from the "clinical" to the "social" dimensions of care, to include vital human rights aspects such as functioning, disability and social inclusion (Inge Petersen et al. 2011). The MHPF already underline these ideals (National Department of Health 2013), but provinces are required to formulate and operationalise area-specific plans in line with this policy. This is an important consideration towards creating contextually-sensitive mental health services, as uniform policy implementation may not adequately accommodate the variations of state and non-state service providers, nor the marked differences between rural and urban settings (Ermien Van Pletzen et al. 2013).

Conclusion

The fractured nature of mental health service provision in LMICs persists, despite significant progress during the past decade. This study underlines crucial gaps in organisational integration among mental health service providers, as well as pointing to complex dynamics among state and non-state sectors in health care provision. Many mental health service gaps were touched upon, including fragmented services, low engagement between partners, and hospital-centric care. Power remains a key consideration towards better understanding how policies unfold in different contexts and among different actors. The coordination and collaboration explored here require inputs from mental health service users and their families, a substantial missing piece in including the voice of policy beneficiaries and building towards better care continuity. These complexities can only be comprehended through a lens of plurality, and require evidence-based, rigorous research. Ultimately, the window of opportunity in terms of the global, regional and national momentum gained during the past decade towards building public mental health services in LMICs should be grasped in its entirety.

Note

1 This chapter has previously been published in *Health Policy and Planning*.

4 Collaboration between the state and civil society

An uneasy coalition

Introduction

In the previous chapter, a mapping of the mental health system was undertaken, by illustrating mental health service networks in a South African district. However, in reality the borders between state and non-state actors are far from clear. In this chapter, we focus on a particularly important, if neglected, dimension of mental health services: the complex and highly politicised relationship between the State and CSOs. Though the focus is on CSOs that are involved in mental health care, it is important to understand this loose subspecialty in terms of the broader nature of State-CSO relations in the post-apartheid period. Using a single term to describe organisations that are inherently varied, can hide the plurality that has become a central feature of CSOs. However, this plurality should be taken as a key indicator of democratic growth:

> [We adopt] a definition of civil society that celebrates its plurality. It recognizes that the set of institutions within this entity will reflect diverse and even contradictory political and social agendas. As a result state-civil society relations will reflect this plurality. Some relationships between civil society actors and state institutions will be adversarial and conflictual, while others will be more collaborative and collegiate. This state of affairs should not be bemoaned. Instead, it should be celebrated since it represents the political maturing of South African society.
>
> (Habib 2005, p. 672)

Post-apartheid policy contexts shaping CSO activities

The roles, responsibilities, identities and activities of CSOs were substantially altered during South Africa's democratising period, where a host of structural, legislative and policy changes took effect. The civil society domain was very much enabled and constrained by the "brave new world" constructed by business and the state (Heinrich 2001). The apparent wave of neoliberal-inspired social policy in many young democracies can very much be conceptualised in terms of Bourdieu's "bureaucratic field", a mechanism that acts like a sphere that influences the motivations and practices of CSOs (Janse van Rensburg et al. 2018), who "attach themselves to new procedures designed to meet the disciplinary demands of the neoliberalizing bureaucratic field" (Woolford & Curran 2012, 48).

The bureaucratic field acts as a prism that refracts economic neoliberal policy, affecting almost all aspects of society (Wacquant 2009a); "the working of the economic system here not only "influences" the rest of society but actually determines it – as in a triangle the sides not merely influence but determine the angles (Polanyi 1977, 14). The neoliberal market-driven ideology of 'lower costs, higher efficiency' that pervaded state power (Žižek 2010), infused South Africa's post-apartheid bureaucratic field and inevitably permeated the ways in which CSOs were structured (Habib 2005). Furthermore, the global hegemony of "poverty reduction" within international development (Ferguson 2015), with significant resource support from international agencies to CSOs, created a system that insisted on measurement and indicators – reigning in and depoliticising CSOs' strategizing capabilities (Mitlin et al. 2007). Market-led relations and increasing commercialisation threatened the core values of the CSO sector: corporate human resourcing rather than volunteerism; financial accountability rather than community accountability; and dependence rather that autonomy. This unfolded against the backdrop of key policy and legislative shifts.

The Constitution of the Republic of South Africa (South African Government 1996) has been, in many ways, the lynchpin of post-apartheid re-building and development. Importantly, it presented the new African National Congress (ANC) government with a substantial amount of symbolic capital, rendering the state into "hope generating machine" (Müller 2014, 41). While the human rights ethos of the Constitution acted as a blueprint for succeeding legislation and policy, the ANC had to balance socio-economic transformation in step with the global milieu during the 1990s, on the one hand, and social justice and the restoration of entitlements, on the other (Sitas 2010). In this vein, the Reconstruction and Development Programme (RDP) was particularly significant, aiming to address colonial and apartheid-era injustices by targeting poverty and unequal social service distribution with a social-democratic approach (Karriem & Hoskins, 2016). The expansion of health and social services during this period is significant – health care is a strategic public good, and a key source of contestation: "Health systems frame and either legitimate or de-legitimate the very nature and competence of the state. States that cannot ensure health care, lose their legitimacy" (Mackintosh 2013).

Health and social development were especially prominent in RDP-led gains during the first years of democracy. This included the provision of free PHC to vulnerable groups; the implementation of an essential drugs programme; greater parity in district-level health expenditure; a clinic building and upgrading programme; expanding welfare benefits to those in need; and a revitalisation and construction of public hospitals (Harrison 2009; Van Rensburg and Engelbrecht 2012). Yet, it quickly became apparent that the RDP was in trouble; this became evident in the missing of targets of the first few years of implementation, as well as underspending and allegations of corruption. The RDP also suffered from ambiguity, some perceiving it as a radical socialist transformation, while others seeing it as an anti-poverty programme (Blumenfeld 1997). Weak power and bureaucratic obstructions in implementing the RDP across various national departments further hamstrung its outcomes (Karriem & Hoskins 2016). Ultimately, apart from selected quantitative progress, the RDP did not qualitatively improve the plight of vulnerable populations such as PLWMI. Van Zyl Slabbert (2006, 102) spoke to the core of the RDP's legacy: "In whichever way we look at it, we will measure the success of our transition by the demonstrable improvement in the quality of life at the local level. That is where we live every day".

Following the RDP, the Growth, Employment, and Redistribution (GEAR) policy was introduced in 1996. The apparent dramatic shift from a somewhat Keynesian RDP to a neoliberal GEAR has been well described (Bond 2005; Karriem & Hoskins 2016; Nattrass 1996; Peet 2002; Terreblanche 1999; Visser 2005). In many respects, GEAR reflected global neoliberal forces at work during the time (International Monetary Fund and World Bank influences in many developing states), prioritising deregulation, privatisation and market dynamics above redistribution and social justice (Harvey 2005). Importantly, GEAR provided a fertile environment for the proliferation of private hospital groups and privatisation of mental health services, adding impetus to an already fractured, unequal and dualistic health system. Perhaps the most striking indication of the ideological shift from the RDP to GEAR was the transfer of oversight power from the presidency to the Ministry of Finance, cementing the transformation from "growth through redistribution" to "redistribution through growth" (Karriem & Hoskins 2016). Adding to calls for increased state-civil society collaboration in the ANC Health Plan and White Paper for the Transformation of the Health System in South Africa, the Non-Profit Organisations Act 71 of 1997 created a formal, legal structure for such relations. Specifically, the Act allows for CSOs to register as public benefit organisations, and set standards of governance, transparency and accountability by offering inducement rather than penalty in creating structure for voluntary registration (South African Government 1997.

As discussed in the previous chapter, the narrative of collaborations across state and non-state divides, as well as across sectors, has been firmly put in centre stage by the introduction of the ambitious, state-driven National Health Insurance (NHI) scheme. A notable feature of this project has been a combative tone between state and private care sectors. Throughout his tenure, the Minister of Health spearheading the NHI Dr Aaron Motsoaledi, took a firm public stance against a perceived frivolous and unjust private sector, adopting war language and casting the stand-off as an ideological battle rather than a pragmatic economic one. Probably due to coinciding with Barack Obama's introduction of the Affordable Health care Act in the United States at the same time, a similar discourse of socialist versus free market medicine was deployed. Alex van den Heever, a prominent voice of critique against the NHI proposals, noted that the Green Paper on a Policy on National Health Insurance contains factually incorrect information that deliberately inflate the public-private health care system discrepancies in South Africa (van den Heever 2011). Indeed, the public-private divide in rhetoric regarding the reasons for and need to curb private sector labour costs and decrease social inequality persists, and will likely continue to haunt the broader discourse of universal coverage.

The roles and responsibilities of CSOs

Finding a vocation in the New South Africa

CSOs have taken up a critical role in promoting the well-being of South African communities, both before and after attaining democracy, especially in delivering health-related services (van Pletzen, Zulliger, Moshabela, & Schneider 2014). We have alluded to the service delivery role of CSOs in mental health care provisioning, but there are some key considerations that will need to be unpacked in order to understand and appreciate the political economy relations that emerge during collaborative activities with the state. As mentioned in the previous chapter, there are several organised efforts driven by Afrikaner nationalist-type Christianity that have been in place in different scope and size for the past century. Up until 1994, various CSOs took up a strong advocacy role, by opposing and resisting the apartheid state using a range of strategies. Black Sash is an especially prominent example, and there is a rich history describing the anti-apartheid efforts of civil society (Konieczna & Skinner 2019). In short, a large proportion of CSOs in a singular goal, namely to further the democratic and pro-human rights ideals leading up to the 1994 election. After the ANC won these elections, CSOs found themselves in a peculiar position – now that democracy has been achieved, what is their role? To what ideal can they now hitch their wagons?

Adam Habib has described this transition well and remains an authority on civil society during the transition from apartheid, commenting in 2005 that the adversarial-collaborative divide between pro and anti-apartheid CSOs gradually dissolved as a racial split in civil society became more blurred (Habib 2005). He describes the development of CSOs in two movements, namely the anti-apartheid mobilisation during the 1980s liberalisation movement, funded by foreign backers and an aided by an injection of advocacy-minded students and graduates from 1970s political struggle, and the post-1994 democratisation period, where CSOs had to adapt and change to participate in a new environment. Importantly, CSO resources were recast in this period, and many CSOs were absorbed into new state institutions and functions

(James Ferguson [2006] noted that the "N" in "NGO" increasingly fell away in Southern Africa's post-apartheid era). Others, especially those involved in mass movements, reorganised themselves to compliment state functions by partnering with government departments to provide social development and welfare activities. Yet another group of CSOs held fast to a liberal approach, positioning themselves as independent watchdogs over the newly formed state (Habib & Taylor 1999). Indeed, while CSOs played a vital part in changing South Africa's socio-political landscape, "In the process, civil society has itself been remolded" (Habib 2005, p. 677). Their role changed from stark opposition to government, to finding new ways in which to engage with government (Community Agency for Social Enquiry, Planact, & Africa Skills Development 2008). In this new role, CSOs had to fulfil three essential democratisation roles, namely to act as "schools of democracy", to help mitigate societal conflict, and to act as voices for the poor and marginalised in the higher echelons of governance and policymaking (Heinrich 2001). These ideals were expedited towards the end of the 1990s, when the honeymoon period for the young democracy started to wane, amidst mounting pressure on the ANC to deliver on its ambitious promises.

Oversight and advocacy

Not only had the ANC underperformed in service delivery, but trade unions – a vital part of the anti-apartheid struggle – was thought to sell out the people by participating in the tripartite alliance. During this time, the advocacy voice of large CSOs seemed to be relatively quiet, having to get used to walking a middle path between taking a position of critiquing government and receiving funding from and collaborating with government. Many CSOs subsequently found it difficult to straddle the roles of partner and critical evaluator (Community Agency for Social Enquiry et al. 2008). However, with the now infamous post-1998 Mbeki presidency's AIDS denialism, there was once again a common enemy for CSOs to focus on. Mbeki was tasked to "build the nation" that was liberated by Mandela but inherited serious challenges. A chief one was a growing concern over ANC corruption and cronyism (a coat that the ANC would never really be able to shed, especially given Zuma's "lost decade"). The corruption challenge was perhaps best illustrated by the Sarafina II debacle, which has to some extent become a Watergate-type syntax for ANC corruption, revived in recent times during Nkosazana Dlamini-Zuma's resurgence in parliamentary politics.

The Mbeki government's handling of the HIV/AIDS epidemic has today almost legendary status, a near-perfect example of how to not govern an infectious disease. While the infamous peddling of herbal remedies on an international stage was certainly a memorable (and farcical) feature of the response, there are five main dimensions that contributed to the disastrous anti-AIDS stance (Fourie 2006). The proliferation of human rights-inspired legislation passed under the Mandela years created an enabling environment for the pursuit of individual rights to care, and "a culture of legislation and litigation" became the norm during the Mbeki AIDS stance. From very early on, the government response to AIDS was draped in anti-intellectualism, rooted in Mbeki's suspicion of the causal links between HIV and AIDS. Access to drugs that prevent mother-to-child transmission of HIV became a key battleground for civil society to challenge AIDS policy. Furthermore, the monetisation of AIDS become more pressing, as the economic costs (always a persuasive argument) of AIDS compared to a public response started to emerge in the prevailing discourses around the issue. Finally, a reappraisal of the structural drivers of HIV/AIDS emerged, very much rooted in a rhetoric of culture and race (Fourie 2006). These features of the state's AIDS response created fertile ground for the establishment and growth of the Treatment Action Campaign, a CSO that ultimately would define health activism in the new millennium and lead the civil society charge in the battle against the state's denialism and inaction. Since its inception in 1998, the TAC relied on a combination of protest, legal action and social mobilisation to pressure Mbeki's government as well as large pharmaceutical companies to enable access to life-saving antiretroviral drugs. A powerful asset that the TAC had during this time was a large membership of passionate, young African women, many of whom were openly HIV-positive. The organisation remains at the forefront of health activism today, and continue to lobby for improved health care access for the poor and marginalised. However, where issues such as HIV, gender-based violence, and access to housing and municipal services have been strongly grounded in a spirit of activism and counterpressure, civil society involved in mental health care seem to have been much more docile, rather focusing on the immediate pressures of service delivery. Indeed, activism in the non-communicable disease sphere of civil society has tended lobby for prioritisation by using science as a motivating factor; HIV activist used social justice, litigation and even moral arguments to apply pressure for change. CANSA's anti-tobacco campaigns, SAFMH's depression prioritisation campaigns and the Heart & Stroke Foundation South Africa relies heavily on research and scientific reasoning to get their messages out into the public and political spheres, but crucially lack the tools of mass mobilisation and aggressive politics to affect change (Ndinda, Chilwane, & Mokomane 2013). However, it should be noted that HIV activism was also somewhat supported by a global enabling environment through increased funding and political commitment and will, something that other health priorities often lack. By investing resources in frontline service delivery, away from the limelight of political events, CSOs involved in mental health care are often sidelined in their democratisation role (Heinrich 2001).

Increasingly fuzzy borders of independence

The role of CSOs in public service delivery was once again redefined when the state started, with the advent of Aaron Motsoaledi's reign as health minister and the accompanying renewed drive to establish a National Health Insurance (NHI), to absorb community health workers (CHWs) from CSOs into direct service. Motsoaledi and his team reportedly visited countries where PHC success stories grew; Brazil's Bolsa Familia programme, and Cuba's Family Doctor and Nurse Plan were especially influential in the development of South Africa's PHC Re-engineering Programme. It held the promise of achieving impressive outcomes with less resources, and, importantly, adhered to the strong state-driven socialist roots of ANC policy. Nonetheless, in the contexts of wide-scale shortages in medical practitioners and nurses, the state had to rely on CHWs as the building block for the programme. Before 2010, CHWs were largely employed by CSOs registered with the DoH; the organisations acted as administrative and managerial support, overseeing and compensating CHWs for programme-specific work – the bulk of which related to HIV. With the piloting of PHC Re-engineering, CHWs were taken from CSO's control, to fall under the jurisdiction of provincial health departments, managed by district health offices. In the process, CSOs had to redefine their livelihoods, or perish. Discussions on this transition has focused largely on CHWs themselves, and much less so on the wider impact on civil society (van Pletzen et al. 2014). Not only did CSOs have to content with losing CHWs to the state – a large proportion of civil society expertise in management and finances were lured to state positions by extraordinary salaries, leaving substantial gaps in the abilities of civil society to self-manage and stay afloat (Community Agency for Social Enquiry et al. 2008).

CSOs have found themselves in an increasingly difficult position in recent years, especially those involved in mental health care. They have to carefully tread on the line between service providers for government and voices for the poor and vulnerable. There is a real dilemma for CSOs funded by government – they substantially rely on funding from the DoH and DoSD, and simply cannot afford to bite the hand. Obtaining an official NPO certificate from government has become a defining feature of CSOs – without one, they simply do not exist. They are not recognised as official structures, and cannot tap into the monthly cash stream of the welfare system (Moshabela, Gitomer, Qhibi, & Schneider 2013). Those not registered – like many smaller CSOs providing residential care for people with severe mental illness – rely on the income generated by their beneficiaries' disability grants, needing to keep a low profile. This means operating on the fringes of public scrutiny, until they have accumulated enough capital to develop formal structures and launch publicly, which puts them on the road of getting registered and recognised. Often, such smaller CSOs would use key stakeholders in the local mental health care system, including other, larger NPOs, to help them leverage the capital (economic and otherwise) required to partner with government (Janse van Rensburg 2018; Moshabela et al. 2013). The pressure to survive as an organisation has eroded the need to lobby and pressure those in power, and the TAC remain one of very few examples of how the tightrope can successfully be walked (Community Agency for Social Enquiry et al. 2008). CSOs receive funding from multiple sources, but in the case of mental health care, the main funders are the DoH, who contracts CSOs to provide specific services such as residential geriatric care, and the DoSD, who provides welfare services through in-house delivery, out-contracting, subsidies to CSOs for certain services, and full funding to CSOs to provide services on its behalf (Cornerstone Economic Research 2018). It is exactly in terms of the latter two mechanisms of DoSD funding that a significant conflict between the state and civil society came to pass.

The NAWONGO court case

A decade-long court case between civil society and the state cast a spotlight on the fundamental fissures between these sectors, contesting the boundaries between state and non-state service delivery. It also helps illuminate a particular framing of people living with severe mental illness, a framing that was shot into prominence during the Life Esidimeni crisis. In 2010, a coalition of CSOs – of which the bulk focused on social and welfare services – made an application to the Free State High Court against the MEC for Social Development in Free State, the Head of the Free State Department of Social Development, and the National Minister of Social Development.[1] The coalition, made up of 92 social and welfare CSOs across South Africa (forming the National Association of Welfare Organisations and Non-Governmental Organisations, NAWONGO), Nederduits Gereformeerde Social Services Free State and Free State Care in Action (hereafter collectively referred to as NAWONGO), intended to legally formalise years of conflict with the DoSD regarding subsidies owed for welfare services provided in the public sector. Low payment rates, delays in payment, and a lack of clarity regarding services to be delivered lay at the centre for the application. NAWONGO's demands included that the DoSD should rectify outstanding payments for transfers that have been allocated, and that the policy for compensating non-profit service delivery on behalf of the state be reviewed, especially its funding structure. Critically, the DoSD did not perceive the funding of CSOs to deliver state mandated services as a constitutional obligation, bringing forth the question of state responsibility for the welfare of communities and vulnerable individuals. In a series of judgements from 2010 to 2014, the veil started to lift on the relationship between the state and civil society in the delivering of public mental health care.

2010

In the first judgement, the DoSD acknowledged that the 1 400 CSOs they were funding in the Free State played a critical role in service delivery to the vulnerable, including the elderly, children in poverty, and people with disabilities, services that the DoSD are obligated to provide in line with the Constitution, the Promotion of Equality and Prevention of Unfair Discrimination Act, the

Children's Act, the Older Persons Act, the Child Justice Act, the Prevention and Treatment of Substance Abuse Act, and the Nonprofit Organisations Act. It was also acknowledged that the payments did not cover the full costs of CSO services rendered.

In order to illustrate this discrepancy, the example of child and youth care centres were used. It was estimated that 2000 such centres are needed in the Free State province to fulfil court-mandated placements, and that 320 of the currently available 1085 beds were government-run – the shortfall was picked up by CSOs. The amounts given to CSOs that take care of children in line with the Children's Act fell woefully short of the amount given to state-run institutions, and CSOs were given the impossible task of providing three meals per day at a rate of R11.84 per child under its care. A similar discrepancy emerged in analysing the deficit in financing homeless shelters for children, where the monthly subsidy of R400–R500 per child fell short of the R2000 that was estimated for care. While the exact dimensions and quality of care was not extensively unpacked, it can be assumed that this assumption reflects a minimum amount required to fulfil statutory obligations. This would therefore cover basic needs, but the focus on inputs and outputs as measurement of well-being fall far short of Sen and Nussbaum's ideas on the development of capabilities, agency and citizenship. The judge concluded that the discrepancies between the amount required to provide care to vulnerable people, and the amount actually paid by the DoSD for the outsourcing of such services, amounted to a constitutional breach by violating the rights of the intended beneficiaries of welfare activities. The first judgement was a resounding win by NAWONGO: The DoSD was ordered to revise the Free State Policy on Financial Awards to the Nonprofit Organisations in the Social Development Sector in line with the requirements outlined during the trial; they had to pay outstanding payments to CSOs; and cover the bulk of the legal costs incurred by NAWONGO. Further, due to a lack of confidence in the leadership capabilities of the DoSD to see these tasks through, the court stepped in to supervise these proceedings via a structural interdict. A period of six months was set for the DoSD to revise its policy, including inputs from CSOs. The revisions had to include a recognition that CSOs are providing services that the state was constitutionally obliged to provide, and the method of determining the size of transfers had to be transparent, fair and equitable, with a consideration of additional funds that will need to be sought by CSOs (Van der Merwe 2010).

There are two important considerations that can be gleaned from this first judgement. First, it is apparent that a distinct cost-benefit logic is applied in the court's arbitration approach. It reflects what Polyani called "strongholds of economistic modes of thought" (Polanyi 1977, 18), and will become a central leitmotif in the relations between the state and its non-state partners in public welfare, vividly illustrated in the next chapter during the Life Esidimeni arbitration process. Second, the question of responsibility for the voiceless and marginalised emerged, along with the deeper questions of ethics and justice. Both these considerations would reverberate throughout the conflict, and would be mirrored in other provinces and sectors as well.

2011–2013

Following the first judgement, the DoSD enlisted the services of global auditing giant KPMG to develop a costing model for welfare services and recommendations for the distribution of funds, in addition to rewording the funding policy. The unchallenged inclusion of a company firmly plugged into the global marketplace to fundamentally influence decision-making that is essentially moral, to insert a firm logic of auditing and accountancy as a method to determine investment in human worth, is hugely problematic. The inclusion of KPMG was no doubt an attempt to include an unbiased voice to make the determination of what is economically feasible and fair, though it should be noted that auditing and accountancy as specialised forms of knowledge are far from neutral; as Foucault and his disciples have shown, specialised knowledge is has enormous potential to change every level of society, and has become a key form of power and governance in modern life. The inclusion of KPMG in this arbitration very much points to features of an "audit society"; one where 'the welfare state is increasingly being displaced by the "regulatory" state, and instruments of audit and inspection are becoming more central to the operational base of government' (Power 2000, 114).

An interim report was produced by the KPMG firm, and delivered to NAWONGO for input. This first draft from the DoSD was rejected by the CSOs, who bemoaned the lack of consultation in the development of the draft and the request for an extension for the finalisation and implementation of the revised policy. NAWONGO was not convinced that the KPMG costing model understood the nature of the welfare services that they were supposed to cost. The DoSD proposal that CSOs should also contribute to the costs of services they are delivering on behalf of government was also rejected, as was the assumption that CSO budgets as designated by Treasury were set and unchangeable. Importantly, the interim proposal suggested that the existing CSO funding budget be re-distributed, rather than increasing the budget. That was to be achieved by using the KPMG costing model to calculate the service costs of CSOs. The method was summed up by the presiding judge over the case as follows (Van der Merwe 2011, Sections 8–9):

> Having determined the total annual service cost per NPO, the aggregate of the funding cost of all the NPO's can be determined. The next step is to determine which NPO's can reasonably contribute to their funding costs and to what extent. On the basis that the total NPO funding costs exceed the budget available to the department to fund the NPO's, a formula is proposed which in its simplest form can be stated as:
>
> $x = (A - B) \div C$

> In this formula A is the total annual costs of the services provided by the NPO's calculated as described above, B is the total annual budget available to the department for the funding of these services provided by the NPO's and C is the total own funds of the NPO's reasonably available to contribute to the services provided by the NPO's. When x is multiplied by 100, it provides the percentage that each NPO that is able to contribute to the cost of the services provided by it, is to contribute from the amount reasonably available from own funds to contribute thereto. Thus, if A is R100 million, B is R60 million and C is R50 million, x will be 0.8. When multiplied by 100 the result is 80%. Therefore, an NPO that has funds reasonably available to contribute to the cost of the services provided by it, will be required to contribute 80% of those available funds.

NAWONGO contested this proposal, claiming that the DoSD wanted CSOs to make up shortfalls beyond their capabilities (as estimated by the DoSD). The draft proposal was negotiated in court, leading up to the second judgement in 2011. In this judgement, the judge noted that there are deficiencies between the proposed policy revision and the costing methods employed, and the way in which the percentage covering shortfalls will be calculated were unclear. The revised version still put the responsibility of caring for the vulnerable on the shoulders of CSOs when the DoSD budget is insufficient, which goes against the spirit of the first judgement and does not solve the core dispute. The court therefore found that the revision does not comply with the first judgement, and ordered the development of a new revised policy, with closer consultation with CSOs, and that the state was liable for paying NAWONGO's legal costs (Van der Merwe 2011).

Following this judgement, KPMG conducted a detailed costing exercise of all different types of welfare services provided by CSOs, concluding that – even at a minimum threshold – the total costs provided by CSOs in the Free State province in 2011–2012 amounted to R1.15 billion, far more than the R342 million budgeted by the DoSD for this purpose. This accounted for services rendered, and do not include the services that were not provided as obliged by law. As a matter of solution, KPMG offered five options of funding to the DoSD, each with its own consequences for funding. The allocation approaches were underwritten by a prioritisation process, which relied on a method of fund allocation according to predetermined criteria to decide which programmes are more important than others. Also, the prioritisation relied on services that, according to legislation, *must* be rendered and *may* be rendered. These processes led to a ranking of programmes in line with the following five allocation methods (Cornerstone Economic Research 2018):

1. Prioritisation by Programme Only – prioritising according to adoptions, day care etc.

2. Prioritisation by Programme and Responsibilities – adding an additional dimension such as medical care and residential care.
3. Prioritisation by Programme and Expense Type – adding an additional dimension such as personal costs, overheads.
4. Prioritisation by Programme and Necessity Level – adding levels of full, partial and non-necessities.
5. X-factor Only – adding CSO contributions to address insufficient budget; can be used in combination with options 1–4 if needed.

These suggestions were part of a comprehensive analysis delivered by the DoSD to the court in 2012, leading to a third hearing and judgement in 2013. Going into the hearing, NAWONGO still were not satisfied with the revised policy, arguing that breaches with constitutional and legal obligations were still in place. The DoSD admitted that they did not have the budget to sufficiently compensate the whole range of services offered by CSOs in line with the policy requirements. As a remedy, the DoSD proposed to rank, by programme, the services that they were constitutionally and statutorily obliged to provide; decide necessary, partial and non-necessary costs in each programme; apply inflation-adjusted benchmark costs as determined by KPMG; consider reasonable abilities of CSO to fund-raise; all of which will contribute to the final determination of how much the DoSD can compensate CSOs for services rendered. The DoSD seemed to stall; they acknowledged that they did not have the budget to cover services completely but was hoping that the strategy proposed would ultimately lead to full coverage. NAWONGO objected to the revised approach, stating a lack of consultation, vagueness in KPMG's costing model in terms of what exactly would be covered, and a fear that attempts to cover all services with a limited budget would be spreading funding too thin to offer appropriate assistance. Simply put, similar issues remained from the first judgement. Additionally, mistakes in the KPMG calculations were pointed out, and the DoSD admitted to discrepancies in the revised policy. However, even with changes, the judge still remarked that the improvements to the revised policy is irrelevant if it is still unconstitutional as per the previous two judgements. The proposed allocation model was deemed to be a deficit-sharing model, and, importantly, the power to decide what was essential and what was not fell on the DoSD. Consequently, none of the programmes could be funded to its full requirements, CSOs could not predict how much funding they would receive for each programme, as transfers would depend on the size of the provincially allocated budget. Again, the DoSD were instructed by the court to revise their policy, and had to consult further changes with NAWONGO within 15 calendar days. With their recommendations included, the next revision needed to be submitted to the court to check whether it complies with the Constitution within 60 days from the judgement. Again, the order was made that NAWONGO's costs needed to be covered (Cornerstone Economic Research 2018).

2014 and aftermath

Commenting on the third revision of the DoSD policy during the 2014 judgement, the judge summarised and addressed the core objections from NAWONGO to the latest version by focusing on the following points:

1. A lack of consultation
2. Insufficient funds made available to CSOs that will result in many vulnerable people being deprived of support
3. Little to no progressive realisation of rights
4. Some elements are still unconstitutional
5. Removal of selected expenses from core costs were perceived to be unreasonable and arbitrary
6. The determination of CSO contributions to service funding were arbitrary
7. The revision discriminates between CSOs and state-owned service providers

The judge considered each of these concerns, and ultimately was satisfied that the third revision of the policy is compliant with the first two judgements. The third revised Policy on Financial Awards to the Nonprofit Organisations in the Social Development Sector was therefore deemed in line with the constitutional and statutory obligations of the DoSD. The NAWONGO judgements held significant consequences for the funding of CSO activities in South Africa, and the next step was to determine to what extent provincial departments would be able to uphold the determinisations of this revised policy.

In 2017, the Government Technical Advisory Centre of the National Treasury Department put out a tender for consultants to undertake a Performance and Expenditure Review (PER) of the cost implications of funding CSOs following the NAWONGO court judgements. A report was subsequently produced by Cornerstone Economic Research, with some sombre findings (Cornerstone Economic Research 2018).

The key objective of the analysis was to explore the fiscal considerations for provincial social development departments to scale up from subsidising CSO services to funding CSO services on its behalf, with respect to key welfare services (including a standard programme of assisting people with disabilities which, relevantly, includes people with severe mental illness). In terms of context, the report suggested that, in general, provincial funding for social welfare services were relatively low at 2.3% of the total annual budget. Figures from Treasury showed that, between the 2012/2013 and 2016/2017 financial years, spending from provincial DoSD rose by 9.7% per annum, from R12 billion to R17.8 billion. Over the same period, provincial DoSD's welfare spending increased by 7.5% per annum, from R8.6 billion to R11.5 billion. However, in terms of transfers to CSOs for service provisioning, the increase was 5.2% per annum, from R3 billion to R3.7 billion. Interestingly, in the Free

State – the epicentre of the NAWONGO court battle – the provincial government reduced CSO funding from 162 million in 2013/2014 to R151 million in 2015/2016, contrary to the national trend of increasing funding flows to CSOs. The report further showed that the role of CSOs in the social development sector was substantial, given that 36.6% of the 2016/2017 provincial budget – R6.5 billion – was transferred to CSOs, albeit with wide variety across services according to province (Cornerstone Economic Research 2018). This mirrors the wide variations across provinces in DoH mental health care capacity and delivery as highlighted ealier (Lund, Kleintjes, Kakuma, & Flisher 2010).

The NAWONGO PER review essentially updated and used the KPMG "Combined Costing and Allocation Model" from the NAWONGO case to cost provincially funded CSO services. The main findings suggest that, for the 30% of services that could be included in the costing analysis, there is a 74% funding gap across provinces, amounting to R3.14 billion. This analysis was extrapolated to the remaining 70% of services that could not be included in the analysis (due to a lack of beneficiary data), according to three scenarios: High (worst case scenario), meaning it assumes the highest percentage funding gap per costed service; Medium, meaning that a weighted average percentage gap per costed service is assumed; and Low (best case scenario), meaning it assumes the lowest percentage funding gap for a costed service. The national average costing amounts and calculated funding gaps are summarised in Table 4.1. Accordingly, there is a range in the average funding gap from 48.4% in line with the Low scenario (R3.5 billion), to 88.6% in the High scenario (R29.1 billion). The analysts lean towards the Medium scenario though, suggesting that it is the most robust – this suggests a funding gap of 71% (R9.2 billion).

The main findings of the report were illustrated and disseminated in poster format (Figure 4.1), which also highlighted main recommendations: Develop a long-term strategy to prioritise social welfare services; develop service funding standards for such services; develop and implement a policy for CSO funding in line with the NAWONGO judgements; standardise welfare names and services for improved expenditure reporting; and routinely gather provincial-level information on welfare service providers, both government and non-government (Cornerstone Economic Research 2018). It should be noted that, while the NAWONGO judgements set legal precedent, it could not – due to separation of the state and the court powers – decide policy. The 2014 judgement noted that the court is in no position to judge the merits of a policy, only its legality (Van der Merwe 2014). However, the NAWONGO PER report was a strategic call by Treasury, and perhaps another step towards the formalisation of state and CSO collaboration regarding the delivery of certain services to people with severe mental illness.

An important consideration in this process towards deciding policy is the influence of economic reasoning in shaping public responses to social welfare in broad, and mental health care in particular. Mental health care is not a recognised programme on its own in the DoSD. An arbitrary line is drawn

Table 4.1 Main findings from the NAWONGO PER analysis

Total transfers to CSOs	*High Scenario*	*Medium Scenario*	*Low Scenario*	*Calculated costing result*			*Calculated funding gap*		
	Highest % funding gap for costed service	*Weighted average % funding gap for all costed services*	*Lowest % funding gap for a costed service*	*High scenario*	*Medium scenario*	*Low scenario*	*High scenario*	*Medium scenario*	*Low scenario*
3,739,356	-88.6%	-71.1%	-48.3%	32,801,293	12,919,733	7,235,298	-29,061,937	-9,180,377	-3,495,943

Source: Cornerstone Economic Research 2018.

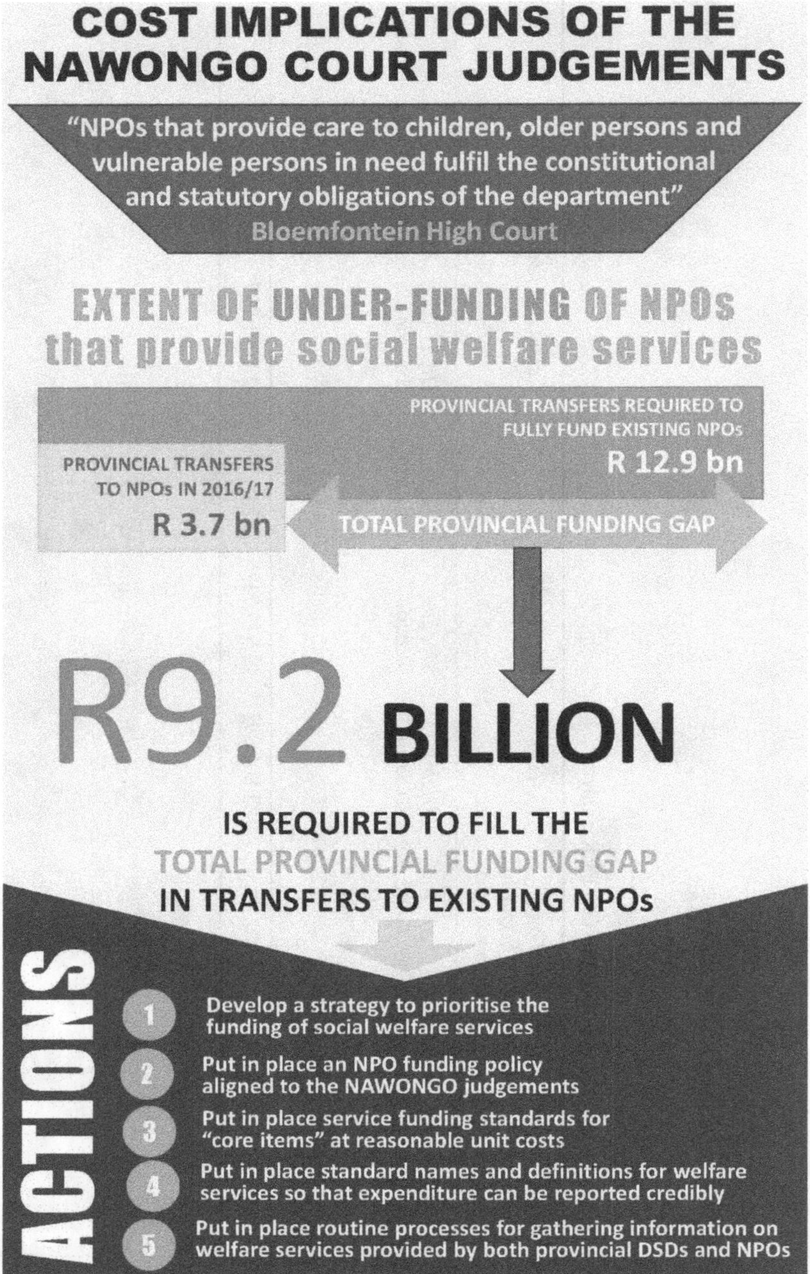
COST IMPLICATIONS OF THE NAWONGO COURT JUDGEMENTS
"NPOs that provide care to children, older persons and vulnerable persons in need fulfil the constitutional and statutory obligations of the department"
Bloemfontein High Court
EXTENT OF UNDER-FUNDING OF NPOs that provide social welfare services
PROVINCIAL TRANSFERS REQUIRED TO FULLY FUND EXISTING NPOs
R 12.9 bn
PROVINCIAL TRANSFERS TO NPOs IN 2016/17
R 3.7 bn
TOTAL PROVINCIAL FUNDING GAP
R9.2 BILLION
IS REQUIRED TO FILL THE
TOTAL PROVINCIAL FUNDING GAP
IN TRANSFERS TO EXISTING NPOs
ACTIONS
1 Develop a strategy to prioritise the funding of social welfare services
2 Put in place an NPO funding policy aligned to the NAWONGO judgements
3 Put in place service funding standards for "core items" at reasonable unit costs
4 Put in place standard names and definitions for welfare services so that expenditure can be reported credibly
5 Put in place routine processes for gathering information on welfare services provided by both provincial DSDs and NPOs

Figure 4.1 Cost implications of the NAWONGO court judgements (Government Technical Advisory Centre, 2018).

between mental illness and disability (the contours of which were highlighted in Chapter 1), and divided between DoH and DoSD. While this line can be made more explicit during institutionalisation in hospitals, it becomes increasingly blurry when care is shifted to community settings, and here we move from a biomedical to an economistic lens. In this way, the relationship between state departments and CSOs should be viewed in terms of the neoliberal-inspired policy structured put in place as touched on at the beginning of the chapter. The increased managerialism in the governance of CSO activities, exemplified in the ways in which the care of people with severe vulnerabilities are reduced to auditing figures in court, where the consideration of subjective needs and experiences of those served are cast aside, are key indicators for a particular approach to governance. In this approach, accounting, auditing and management techniques enable a marketization of public services, allowing for the breaking away from central control and the "inscripting" of expertise-driven governance (Rose 1996a). Here, a calculative technology permeates thought, creates new visibilities of profit and loss, and links private decisions and public objectives through knowledge (Miller & Rose 2008; Rose & Miller 2010b), and cuts across government departments, private sectors and CSOs (Miller 2001). The power of calculations that underwrite the costs associated with the care of individuals within a specific population group lies within its ability to "translate diverse and complex processes into a single financial figure" (Miller 2001, 381). The prevalence of an 'economic machine' that creates structures that dominate through implanting calculating practices, fiscal regimes and financial regulation (Rose 1996a) has then, against the neoliberal turn in post-apartheid South Africa, significantly shaped the governance of mental illness. This cost-benefit economic rationale comes into conflict with core values – referred to by Steven Lukes as incommensurable values – that "resist cost-benefit analysis, where the very idea measuring in order to compare the values of alternative outcomes seem inappropriate" (Lukes 2008, 113). The overly materialist perceptive applied by the court, along with the assumption a revised policy would clear up any issues of fairness and discrimination, is summed up by the judge during the first judgement (Van der Merwe 2010):

> The applicants placed much emphasis on the disparity in funding referred to above and argued that the policy and its implementation amount to unfair discrimination. I do not find it necessary to deal with the question of equality and unfair discrimination. If the policy is redrafted or adjusted in accordance with what is stated above, there should be no question of unfair discrimination.

While we can apply this lens in retrospect, it does not change the effects that the NAWONGO events had, and might continue to have, on mental health care reform.

What do the NAWONGO events mean for mental health care?

It is assumed that the NAWONGO PER report included social welfare services to people with severe mental illness, mostly under the programme of Protected Workshops for people with disabilities. The authors reflected that the very large funding gaps in this area are significant (Cornerstone Economic Research 2018, 29):

> Indeed, so significant that it raises the question whether the content of the protective workshop service costed for the Free State is equivalent to what the provincial DSDs in other provinces are currently funding NPOs to provide? Again, we lack the data to address this, though it should be reiterated that the discrepancy in costs and transfers highlights the need for standard service definitions to guide both the funding and the provision of services.

This point is critical for our discussion here. What exactly do these services entail? This was briefly outlined in the previous chapter, though the exact scope of and nature of services rendered remain relatively undocumented. Lund and Flisher (2009) described community-based mental health care in South Africa in an influential typology, that would ultimately inform the MHFP. It involved a grouping of services according to three types of facilities:

- Type A includes outpatient and emergency services, that include PHC facilities, mobile facilities, community health centres and hospital outpatient and emergency wards.
- Type B includes residential care facilities such as boarding houses, halfway houses and group homes.
- Type C includes day care facilities that offer sheltered employment, independent living, home-based care, social support and recreational support.

While these services are offered in many South African settings, it is – as mentioned in the previous chapter – much less clear-cut and more disordered in reality. This fragmentation especially becomes apparent when one attempts to disentangle the services provided by state services, non-state services, and where these overlap and how. Studies employing social network analysis have added value here, though in limited scope. A 2014 study employed a dual coding to categorise CSOs delivering health services, in terms of its capital (well-resourced, moderately resourced, poorly resourced) and in terms of service orientation (direct services such as psychosocial support, developmental services such as training and mentoring activities in communities, and activist services such as increasing community awareness of rights and access to care). By applying this typology to three districts in South Africa, the study found that well and moderately resourced CSOs were more likely to have a developmental and activist orientation in addition to service orientation, and these sources of capital were largely concentrated in urban areas. In rural areas, CSOs with much less resources, and mostly oriented to deliver services, were more present. These CSOs were also less likely to have strong ties with activist organisations, suggesting less voice in the public sphere in terms of policy, prioritisation and funding decisions (van Pletzen et al. 2014). The disparities suggested in this study was confirmed by another social network analysis, focused on mental health care in a South African district. Here, a wide variety of CSOs were identified providing different forms of mental health care, with different E. degrees of connection to state services. Smaller, less resourced CSOs were also much more on the periphery of the network. Services delivered included residential care, psychosocial counselling, social services, assistance with grant processing, and substance abuse rehabilitation (Janse van Rensburg, Petersen et al. 2018). However, CSOs tend to respond to their environments and perceived needs (which is, after all, a strength), meaning that they often provide services outside of their formal scope, and would often provide whatever services are required by an individual in need. In this way, there are well-connected CSOs in areas such as Cape Town, Johannesburg and Pretoria, that provide structured residential care, with additional day care, basic medical care, education, protective workshops, and counselling, drawing from government funding, private donations, family payments, and by taking a portion of beneficiaries' disability grants. These organisations are often relatively large and well networked, with strong fundraising capabilities. Importantly, they are often registered as official service providers by the DoH, DoSD or, in some instances, by both. This comes with a substantial administrative burden, and requires inspections by government. The basis for the standards of these inspections are unclear, however; CSOs offering residential care are often measured in terms of the National Health Act as "health facilities" – this is not appropriate nor feasible. Some mask their standards by following standards for old age homes. Dedicated, appropriate standards for the regulation of residential and other CSOs are still not in place, despite repeated calls for the development of such norms and standards, including by the NAWONGO PER report. On the other side of the spectrum, there is a group of CSOs that also provide residential care, though in a much more basic fashion. Often located in areas of socioeconomic deprivation, where families cannot afford contributing monthly payments for care, where little fundraising capacity exists, and little to no support from the state and business sector. These organisations generally are not registered at the DoH or DoSD, and therefore receive no formal funding and, critically, no oversight. They remain invisible to health system analysis, because they tend to not appear on government lists of CSOs. Some respond to perceived needs in the community for care for people with severely disabling conditions by starting care homes. While their intentions might be relatively altruistic at the beginning, these organisations often slide into environments that are unfunded, with woefully little expertise, resources and support to care for a population of people that have advanced and complex needs. This often translates into houses filled with beds and/or mattresses, feeding tenants basic meals and helping them to get to a local clinic if required. A key function adopted by these organisations are also to help ensure that their tenants receive their monthly disability grants, which becomes the bulk of income for the daily running of the operation (Janse van Rensburg 2018). Perhaps the most critical oversight in South Africa's post-apartheid mental health system reforms has been neglecting the roles of CSOs, at both ends of the spectrum. A strong focus on developing mental health care in state-run facilities has been driven at the cost of disregarding actual and potential service capabilities of civil society, and provinces have both failed to establish proper intersectoral linkages between departments, and to formally incorporate CSOs into service delivery. The latter means mapping out all CSOs (both registered and non-registered), strategically engage with these CSOs to standardise service packages and including service, developmental and activist oriented partners in planning and service delivery. The inaccuracy and inadequacy of the present mapping of these critical resources are critical barriers in systems reform; the development of community-based care is the only option through which our current over-reliance on hospitals and institutionalisation can be remedied (Docrat et al. 2019).

SASSA grants scandal

As mentioned, a key funding source for CSOs providing residential-based mental health care is claiming monthly disability grants from their clients – this can range from a portion, to the full amount. A key player here is the South African Social Security Agency (SASSA), a welfare grant distribution agency under the jurisdiction of the DoSD, established in 2005. It is essentially a state mechanism tasked with distributing monthly welfare grants to support those who are socioeconomically vulnerable. This includes a Child Support Grant; Older Person's Grant; Disability Grant; Grant-in-Aid; Care Dependency Grant; War Veteran's Grant; and Foster Child Grant. In terms of mental health, the Disability Grant involves, at the time of writing, R1 860 per month, paid to qualifying persons. Qualification entails being between the ages of 18 and 59 years old, be declared medically unfit by a registered medical officer, to be renewed annually. In addition, there is a means test of capital worth, and intended beneficiaries need to fall below a certain line of income and wealth. SASSA became embroiled in a major scandal when, on 3 February 2012, the agency handed a payment system contract to Cash Paymaster Services (CPS), a subsidiary of Net1, a global company trading on the NASDAQ and Johannesburg Stock Exchange. In 2013, the Constitutional Court declared this arrangement legally invalid, and ordered SASSA to either re-launch the procurement process or to find alternative means of welfare distribution. SASSA submitted a plan to the Constitutional Court in 2014 to take over the payment of grants itself when the CPS contract ends on 31 March 2017. However, as the deadline of 31 March 2017 loomed closer for the transfer, it became apparent that SASSA would be unable to pay the approximately \$67 million in welfare grants to 17 million single mothers, people living with disabilities and severe mental illness, pensioners, and war veterans (one-third of the population). In February 2017, SASSA acknowledged its failure to meet this deadline (Maregele 2017). Given the possible catastrophic consequences of non-payment, the Court was forced to – under the emergency procurement conditions of the Public Finance Management Act – order SASSA and CPS to continue the unconstitutional arrangement that was in place before, for another 12 months during which the matter should be resolved. The SASSA Crisis was scathingly placed into context by Constitutional Court Judge Johan Froneman in the opening lines of his judgement of a case between Black Sash and the DoSD, SASSA and others (Mogoeng et al. 2017):

> *One of the signature achievements of our constitutional democracy is the establishment of an inclusive and effective programme of social assistance. It has had a material impact in reducing poverty and inequality and in mitigating the consequences of high levels of unemployment. In so doing it has given some content to the core constitutional values of dignity, equality and freedom. This judgment is, however, not an occasion to celebrate this achievement. To the contrary, it is necessitated by the extraordinary conduct of the Minister of Social Development (Minister) and of the South African Social Security Agency (SASSA) that have placed that achievement in jeopardy. How did this come about?*

Eventually, a contract was signed with the South African Post Office (SAPO), providing the struggling agency with a boost of R2.2 billion per annum. This only emerged after several months of negotiation, a key point of contention being the sharing of personal information between agencies.

A particularly important feature of welfare distribution was exposed during this crisis, namely the building of a "techno-financial system" that track and exploit the poor and socially marginalised (Torkelson 2017). Ways to ensure payment fidelity by means of electronic tracking has been a strong consideration of welfare grant processing, ever since its mention in the White Paper for Social Welfare. A principal reason for SASSA's outsourcing of the welfare contract was to consolidate systems and authenticate beneficiaries. AllPay, a major competitor for the contract, claimed that SASSA made last-minute changes to the tender criteria, from requiring mandatory to preferential biometric verification – "proof of life" was therefore required. Further, Net1 created a range of subsidiaries that targeted beneficiaries to market loans (MoneyLine), mobile phone cards (EasyPay Everywhere), electricity and airtime (Manje Mobile), and insurance (SmartLife). In all, it has been estimated that Net1 accrued as much as US\$420 million profits from the SASSA contract in 2016 alone (Torkelson 2017). Ultimately, it should be kept in mind that social protection policies often become gauze that hides the widening wealth disparities and social costs of neoliberal strategizing (Devereux & Solomon 2011; Harris, Eyles, & Goudge 2016). These strategies starts to transpire when looking at an empirical case of mental health governance from the Free State province.

Note

1 The overview of the legal proceedings was gleaned from a very helpful unpublished summary by Debbie Budlender.

5 Governance of state and civil society mental health care collaboration[1]

Introduction

Globally, there is growing urgency to address mental, neurological and substance abuse disorders in integrated, cost-effective ways – especially in low-to-middle income countries (LMICs) (Jack et al. 2014; Ngo et al. 2013; Patel et al. 2007; Patel et al. 2013; Patel et al. 2015; Wainberg et al. 2017; World Health Organization 2008). In South Africa's pluralistic, state-driven health system, close collaboration between public and private mental health service providers is a key strategy in addressing the burden of mental illness (van Rensburg & Fourie 2016). Private (non-state, non-government, or third-sector) organisations are an established and core component of local public service provision. However, research into their dynamics with public entities remains limited (Bovaird 2014). What is known is that the organisation of these relationships unfolds in hierarchies, markets, networks, or – in South Africa's case – hybrid structures of service delivery (Markovic 2017). The inclusion of NGOs and other private partners in health care provision has gained traction due to weakening formal states and the loss of legitimacy in centralised state governance, as well as the gradual acceptance that complex social problems cannot be resolved by the state alone (Donahue 2004).

Similarly, mental illness cannot simply be resolved with pharmacology and psychotherapy, but requires collaboration across services to effectively address its devastating effects on both individuals and communities (Mechanic, Mcalpine, & Rochefort 2014; Millward et al. 2009; Thornicroft & Tansella 2002). Despite increased global efforts to achieve the ideal of comprehensive mental health care by integrating social and health services, success has been mixed (Butler et al. 2008; Butler et al. 2011; Maruthappu, Hasan, & Zeltner 2015; Mechanic 2003). Paradoxically, integrated care initiatives have been plagued by fragmented approaches, across different contexts, health systems, cultural and governance structures, and definitions of key terms (Kodner 2009; Kodner & Spreeuwenberg 2002; Ouwens, Wollersheim, Hermens, & Hulscher 2005). Indeed, collaboration and partnership across the structural and cultural boundaries of siloed approaches has become something of a unicorn, both attractive and seemingly unattainable (Fimreite & Lægreid 2009).

The division between health and social sectors particularly affects socially marginalised people, with chronic conditions including people with mental illness (PWMI) (Nicaise et al. 2013). In South African health care, "operational governance is embedded within and influenced by the organizational and system-level governance arenas", and local service managers are often faced with constraints from broader organisational and system design issues (Scott et al. 2014, p. 67). The failure of national mental health policy implementation on district levels is an effect of decentralised governance to provinces, leading to fractured prioritisation, implementation and monitoring (Draper et al. 2009; Van Rensburg & Engelbrecht 2012a). In such settings, integrated systems of care become even more difficult to achieve (Mechanic 2003).

The fragmentation of care is a real and pressing concern for health systems. In the case of mental illness, the knocking down of the "Berlin Wall" between health and social care has been an persistent challenge (Dickinson & Glasby 2010). Across the past two decades, a wealth of literature has spawned addressing how to break down this wall and create integrated health systems, with governance highlighted as especially critical (D'Amour, Goulet, Labadie, Martín-rodriguez, & Pineault 2008; Janse van Rensburg & Fourie, 2016; Janse van Rensburg et al. 2016; Mitchell & Shortell 2000; Mur-Veeman et al. 2003; Pim Peter Valentijn et al. 2015; Pim P. Valentijn, Schepman, Opheij, & Bruijnzeels 2013). The dynamics of governance mechanisms in collaborative arrangements are crucial in fostering beneficial partnerships (Hill & Lynn 2003), but evidence of the particularities of the governance processes are lacking (Willem & Lucidarme 2014), as are questions on how to effectively govern networks geared towards 'wicked problems' (Cristofoli, Meneguzzo, & Riccucci 2017). Simply put, we cannot expect to begin to understand outcomes before opening up the black box of the social processes of governing public-private collaboration (Brazil et al. 2005). The governance of service delivery networks requires empirical insight into the processes of power and influence (Heen 2009), and herein lies our study focus. In this Chapter we interrogate the relations between state and non-state mental health service providers, in a South African district. Accordingly, the principle aim of this study was to understand the power dynamics in governance processes of district-level public mental health service provision.

Methods

The findings were derived from a larger, mixed methods study that involved social network analysis as well as key informant interviews. As a study of governance dynamics within a geopolitical delineated space, with distinctive units of analysis, this study employed a qualitative single-case embedded design (Yin 2009). From October to November 2015, all 66 public and non-state health facilities providing mental health care in Mangaung Metropolitan District were visited, and social network data were collected. Following initial analysis, pertinent network groupings of public and non-state service

Table 5.1 List of state/non-state mental health collaborations

State facility		*Non-state facility*	
Code	*Services provided in collaboration*	*Code*	*Service provided*
Clinic	Out-patient drug treatment	NGO	Housing, rehab, treatment adherence
Clinic	Out-patient drug treatment	NGO	Social/welfare services, psychotherapy
		NGO	Housing/rehab, treatment adherence
		NGO	Housing/rehab
		NGO	Substance abuse rehab and prevention
		NGO	Housing, treatment adherence
Clinic	Out-patient drug treatment	NGO	Social/welfare services, psychotherapy
Psychiatric hospital	Acute and serious case processing; social/ welfare services	NGO	Social/welfare services, psychotherapy
		NGO	Housing/rehab
Clinic	Out-patient drug treatment	NGO	Housing, treatment adherence
District hospital	Out-patient drug treatment; acute and serious case processing	NGO	Housing, treatment adherence

collaboration were identified for further in-depth analysis (see Table 5.1 for breakdown). These participants were augmented with key informants identified through a snowball sample that involved asking participants to identify influential actors in district-level mental health care (see Table 5.2 for breakdown). 20 semi-structured interviews were conducted in face-to-face settings, yielding 23 hours of discussions. As all participants were fluent in English, all interviews were conducted in English. Interviews were audio recorded, transcribed verbatim, and analysed with the assistance of NVivo10.

A thematic analysis approach was followed, namely, "summative, phenomenological meanings of text ... [that] represent the essences and essentials of humans' lived experiences" were categorised according to a theoretical framework (deductive) and were constructed from repeated reading of the transcripts (inductive) (Saldaña 2014). Pre-determined themes were deductively generated from the Framework for Assessing Power in Collaborative Processes (Purdy 2012). Themes related to health system stewardship emerged inductively during the data analysis process. Three researchers negotiated themes and their content to achieve consensus, and to remove overlap from the data. De-identified direct quotations were used to support thematic categorisation. Participants were informed in writing and verbally of the purpose of

Table 5.2 List of key informant positions and affiliations

Position	*Affiliation*
State	
Senior psychologist	Government department; Specialist hospital
Programme director	Government department
Psychiatrist	Psychiatry outreach team; District hospital
Psychologist	District hospital
Mental health nurse	District hospital
Mental health nurse	PHC clinic
Non-state	
Case worker	Non-profit organisation
CEO	Private for-profit psychiatric hospital
Director	Non-profit organisation

the research, were guaranteed anonymity and confidentiality, and all provided informed consent. All ethical approvals were obtained from the researchers' institution.

Findings

The findings are presented as follows: First, the themes derived deductively from Purdy's Framework for Assessing Power in Collaborative Governance Processes (2012) are presented, according to the processes of collaborative governance in public administration. This includes *Participants*, *Process Design*, and *Content*, presented in terms of different arenas of power. Second, during the analysis several themes emerged inductively from the data, which were merged after negotiation and consensus among researchers. These themes largely related to *Mental health stewardship*, and included the sub-themes *Information and monitoring systems*; *Mental health financing structures*; *Prioritisation*; *Mental health within broader reforms*; and *Strategic leadership*. Finally, limited indications of *Resistance* to governance processes emerged.

Participants

Participants and formal authority

Participation in the district mental health service delivery network was influenced by state health system hierarchy, a key feature of formal authority. Public participants mentioned that they are firmly bound to provincial referral policy that omits non-state service providers. Private participants in turn were cognisant of the importance of adhering to these formal rules. NGOs sought out PHC clinics in their geographical area to access clinical care for clients suffering from mental illness. Public facilities in turn referred people suffering from mental illness for psychosocial aftercare to NGOs. However, the limited service capacities of NGOs in rural areas were perceived by public service participants as constraints to collaboration. NGOs were further heavily dependent on Department of Social Development (DoSD) funding, and Department of Health (DoH) participants seemingly did not engage in this issue, and showed reluctance to operate outside of the DoH governing sphere. Identification documents, welfare grant management and other social support issues were perceived to be within the ambit of NGOs with social workers in their workforce – under the legislative governance of the DoSD. Public participants often chose organisations that provided basic care and housing to collaborate with, in agreements that in some cases spanned several decades. In this vein, old age homes were mentioned to be particularly "useful", since facilities for geriatric care were perceived to be appropriate for the management of mental illness. In an almost complete absence of public substance abuse rehabilitation facilities, several public facilities collaborated with an organisation providing substance use rehabilitation, subsidised by the DoSD for limited beds on a monthly basis. It was made clear though, that the state maintained responsibility for mental health care, as illustrated by the following excerpt:

> *Whether they get funded through grants, or through tax increases, or whatever, the work that NGOs do is the state's responsibility. The only reason that they do it is because they do it on behalf of the state. So you can never financially untie yourself from an NGO.*
>
> (SW_TH)

Participants and resources

Participants varied in their access to resources within collaborative arrangements, demonstrated by the affordances to differing professional backgrounds. The bulk of clinical experts – including psychiatrists, psychologists, mental health nurses, and social workers – were situated in public health facilities, particularly in hospitals. NGOs leveraged occupational therapists at public hospitals in order to complete assessments required for their clients to gain access to welfare grants. The discipline of social work was highlighted as a key mechanism in collaboration between service providers. Social workers' embeddedness in and access to community-based resources was highlighted as a vital point of collaboration with different partners. For example, social workers were valuable role-players in a collaborative arrangement between the public psychiatric hospital and a specialised mental health NGO. Social workers at the hospital served as gatekeepers for the NGO to specialised services, while social workers from the NGO conducted home visits and provided other community-based services for the hospital.

Participants and discursive legitimacy

Discursive legitimacy emerged in terms of the status of participants and the use of coalitions to further interests. There was a sense of distrust in the capacities of public officials to lead mental health care, due to concerns related to corruption and political venality. On the other hand, some public participants were distrustful of NGOs providing mental health care. Others were of the view that NGOs are an essential part of the service delivery network, and opined that "at times it seems as if even we rely on them more than they rely on us really" (PN_PHCC1). Some NGO participants thought that they had special abilities to work with and manage mental illness (especially psychosis), not tied to professional mental health disciplines:

> *We know how to handle them. I think it is my work from the heaven because if I come here and talk to the people with mental (sic), they listen to me.* (CC_NGO1)

NGOs varied widely in terms of resources, with one participant stating "skilled workers equals money, and money is our only drawback" (CC_NGO4). A constrained funding environment resulted in some participants using personal resources to keep their organisations afloat. While some NGOs employed mental health professionals, others focused on providing basic care such as clothing, housing and treatment adherence and were therefore dependent on public facilities for clinical services, as well as public funding. Well-funded NGOs saw themselves as superior to public service providers in terms of quality, cost-effectiveness and efficiency, and one stated that "the state does not have the resources. They don't have the money to keep this massive machine going" (CC_NGO3).

Less well-funded NGOs that provided mental health services were perceived to be struggling not only in attaining human resources, but also financially – especially in contrast to well-funded programs such as HIV. Some public participants revealed a degree of sympathy towards the plight of mental health NGOs in light of little support from DoSD. This status did however afford NGOs the status of champions for the poor and neglected, despite the personal financial constraints faced by workers. NGOs sometimes used strategic partners as a source of power, engaging with influential state actors in order to ensure service delivery. For example, an NGO providing housing, treatment adherence and basic social care to PWMI struck up a relationship with a mental health focal person in a district hospital, giving them access to district mental health meetings and increasing their visibility to PHC clinics in the area. In return, the district hospital viewed the NGO as a halfway house, where PWMI can be managed in terms of treatment adherence.

Less-endowed NGOs suggested they were equal partners with the state. Some public participants echoed this sentiment, although others were less enthusiastic about the status of NGOs providing boarding and treatment support to PWMI. Deeper state engagement in monitoring NGO activities was recommended, with increased involvement of mental health professionals. The legitimacy of both non-state and non-clinical actors was called into question, rooted in a strong belief that public mental health professionals providing care in hospitals are a superior strategy in service delivery. One mental health nurse made it clear that NGOs are "outsiders", supported by the state, suggesting that NGOs are service providers rather than partners. Many public participants had little insight into the services rendered by NGOs and had never visited the premises. This said, one public mental health nurse expressed a desire to visit these NGOs to provide assistance and clinical support, however hospital management made it clear that this responsibility falls beyond the DoH's sphere.

Psychiatrists were identified as particularly powerful in district mental health decision making, due to psychiatry's legitimacy compared to that of social work, psychology, and nursing. In service delivery, the psychiatric hospital was seen as having elevated status, which was amplified as it also served as the base for psychiatric outreach, NGOs mentioned that the bulk of their clients are discharged patients from the psychiatric hospital, suggesting a level of dependency on the hospital for a client base. NGOs also had the status of being an agent conduit for community access, in that public health workers often relied on them to follow-up on patients and assess their living conditions – a responsibility that fell through the cracks between social work in DoH and social work in DoSD. This again illustrated the role of social work in the service network, as these workers created a bridge between public and non-state spheres. A fitting example is the arrangement between the public psychiatric hospital and an NGO run by social workers, where the NGO was used to provide services falling outside the sphere of legitimacy to patients.

Process design

Process design: Formal authority and resources

Collaborative processes were significantly state-owned. This is apparent in the dependence of NGOs on state funding, administrative and legislative support, as well as the hierarchical nature of referral patterns according to levels of public health care. No formal agreements were in place, and collaboration occurred in a piecemeal, informal fashion, dependent on key actors in health facilities to reach out to others in order to extend the scope of care for patients suffering from mental illness. It was expected that NGOs refer patients in need of clinical treatment to public facilities, or in rare cases where patients had appropriate medical insurance, to a private psychiatric institution. Public facilities, in turn, were expected to refer patients to relevant NGOs according to geographical access and specific needs. Expectations between public and private service providers generally depended on the specifics of collaborative relationships. In general, the expectation was that public facilities provide clinical treatment, while NGOs provide different types of social care – including housing, treatment adherence support, psychosocial rehabilitation and psychotherapy, and drug and alcohol rehabilitation. Participants from NGOs frequently visited public facilities while accompanying patients in their care, while public participants rarely ventured out of the public service provision sphere. The responsibility to initiate and foster collaboration with non-state service providers was the state's responsibility, both by public and private participants.

Instances of conflict among NGOs and public facilities emerged in administration of correct paperwork and patients' personal identifying documentation. The importance of this expectation was tied to both NGOs and their clients' dependence on social welfare grants, a procedure that relies heavily on correct documentation. Public participants expected NGOs to bring identification and medical documentation with them during visits, sending NGOs back if documents were absent. Given the processing and governance value of such documentation in health care access, this expectation placed public facilities (with their clinical expertise) in an advantageous position. In turn, NGOs provided information of their services to public collaborators. In one collaborative case, a public psychiatric hospital obtained information on types of therapy and psychosocial support groups available from an NGO, so that they could refer patients accordingly.

Meetings between public and non-state collaborating partners differed substantially, ranging from informal telephonic contact to regular formal face-to-face meetings. The psychiatric hospital offered a yearly catered social as a way of thanking NGOs for their efforts. The most prominent space for contact was a quarterly mental health district forum, held at and paid for by the DoH provincial headquarters. Selected non-state service providers in the service network were invited and participated. While many public participants felt that this meeting proved an opportunity for collaboration, private participants seemed less encouraged about the effectiveness of these meetings. Some went as far as to describe the meetings as political grandstanding, having no clear structure, aims and outcomes, stating:

> *If you look at what is said in Batho Pele [national patient rights charter] that every person has a right, have a right to best health services that he can get. I go to the Free State mental health meetings, where the police and all that sit and then you have to listen to countless promises and whatever, and I just shake my head.*
>
> (CC_NGO3)

Process design and discursive legitimacy

Sectorial fragmentation emerged in district forums, where several siloed meetings related to mental health were held between public and private participants. Some participants took part in a forum for mental health (driven by DoH), some in a forum for NGOs (driven by a NGO coalition), some focused on addiction and rehabilitation (driven by DoSD), and some in a forum focusing on disability (driven by DoSD). The participants did not seem to perceive mental health as a cross-cutting, multifaceted phenomenon, and it was often framed in terms of a medical challenge under the stewardship of the DoH.

Communication about the collaboration processes occurred in some instances via referred patients the patients themselves carrying their own medical information with them. However, the NGO expressed dissatisfaction with the process, as some patients would be referred without notice and little information. Additionally, public PHC clinics also expressed this sentiment, seeing a lack of communication and coordination when NGOs brought their clients for care.

Content

Content and formal authority

Within one public and non-state relationship, there was a mutual expectation that the NGO would provide six weeks of care for patients, after which patients would return to the psychiatric hospital for outpatient care. However, participants from this particular NGO took part in this arrangement somewhat begrudgingly, questioning the fairness of the weight in the division of labour. For more than a decade preceding the interviews, tension had been building between NGOs and the state – specifically the DoSD – based on compensation for social, welfare, and mental health services provided. One NGO made it clear that the care of people suffering from mental illness was the state's responsibility, and that NGOs fill the role of contracted service providers (that had to be used because of the claim that they can provide higher quality, more cost-effective social services):

> *Now the answer is given – it is the state's responsibility, this is said in the Constitution [but] they must prove that they can do the services better and provide cheaper ones. Otherwise, they must use our services.*
>
> (CC_NGO4)

The nature and governance of district-level mental health collaboration was subjected to intense scrutiny, when, more than a decade earlier, Free State-based NGOs formed a national coalition with the purpose of taking the DoSD to court in order to clarify the role and compensation of non-state entities in providing social and behavioural services. The coalition – the National Association of Welfare Organisations and Non-Government Organisations (NAWONGO) – was particularly geared towards providing a stronger position for NGOs in their relationship with the state. Some NGO participants were particularly aware of their precarious position, providing independent civic services on the one hand and becoming service providers who are dependent on the state on the other: "sometimes [they] feel as if they are walking on eggs, you don't want to annoy them because you are afraid of losing your funding" (CC_NGO7). The arbitrary nature of choice of investment into NGOs by the DoSD was questioned, in that they are supposed to fund organisations with the best capacity to provide the services they need. The point was further made that NGOs and government departments cannot work in partnership, due to a perception that the state uses the term to shift responsibility to NGOs.

Unification of NGOs was perceived as providing greater bargaining power and pooled resources for court and legal fees. Thus, unity in the coalition based on alignment to better funding structures was questioned by some participants, given the multitude of different interests voiced by different NGOs – who also essentially are in competition with each other (referred to as "a minefield" by one participant). Following a narrative of economic cost-benefit considerations, sentiments of despondency were raised:

> Look, the court case did result in a small increase in subsidy, but if you look at the bigger picture, the increase that did occur was so minimal. Literally, minimal, and I really don't think that it was worth the effort.
> (CC_NGO7)

> *The problem is, they ultimately negotiated in such a way that we are painted into a corner. The state said: OK, we will pay you what you should get, but then only the first four organisations on the priority list will be subsidised. We would have fallen away to number ten or twelve, and prevention to number 30. So it would have meant that we would receive no subsidy*
> (CC_NGO5)

Content and resources

In the absence of a unified mental health information system, little or no routine information was gathered and shared among service providers. In the public sphere, one of the only indicators gathered by the district health system is the number of new patients. Little evidence emerged that this was used in planning and governance processes. Furthermore, the infrastructural challenges faced by smaller community-based NGOs severely restricted their method and frequency of voice, given that often they did not have a telephone, fax or internet presence, making them dependent on larger NGOs and public mental health actors to access the mental health service network. Information shared among public and private participants mostly involved telephone conversations and email. For instance, a participant at the public psychiatric hospital queried a mental health NGO to follow up on discharged patients requiring additional support, including assistance with financial management, acquiring identification documents, accessing disability grants, and processing curatorship. Some NGOs did not have initial access to the quarterly mental health forum, and were dependent on key public participants to be formally invited. As far as could be determined, the dialogue was led by the DoH, and minutes were not circulated. The bulk of private participants had no knowledge of the existence of a national mental health policy, and therefore did not analyse mental health care according to its strategic parameters. A fractured understanding of institutionalisation emerged. While most public participants voiced that institutionalisation was to be avoided according to public policy, NGOs who specialised in providing housing and basic care framed it rather as a necessity in protecting families from harm, based on their observations:

> *They are beating them. They are beating their mothers, they make so many bad things at home. Their fathers, their families. Their families suffer too much.*
>
> (CC_NGO1)

> *And they assaulted the families and those type of things because the families did not understand from the beginning. The families left them alone and this lead to them for instance being without medication, they guys start using drugs and drink and then they get home and put the house on fire, hit the mom and dad and now everyone is scared, you see?*
>
> (CC_NGO3)

Content and discursive legitimacy

There was a palpable lack of official strategy and awareness about mental illness and approaches to it, across sectors and service providers. Key differences among mental health providers translated into different interpretations of the causes, meaning and approaches to mental illness. As per the scope of this study, the focus was on mood disorders including depression and anxiety. However, throughout data collection it became apparent that the lack of consensus of what mental illness is and how it should be managed would render any attempt to ring-fence the focus of disorders futile. Therefore, participants' differing understandings of mental illness are described, and how these meanings translated into collaboration.

Perceived causes of mental illness included treatment non-adherence, substance abuse, relationship problems, poverty and the stress associated with life in poverty. Several participants noted that mental illness presented in terms of sleeplessness, loss of appetite, and a general sense of worry. It was noted that mental illness is nebulous in nature, not lending itself to easy diagnosis:

> *Because psychiatry is a difficult thing, you cannot see it. Is the guy depressed or not? I can fake depression*
>
> (CC_NGO8)

Some mental health professionals suggested that mental illness presents differently between different cultural and ethnic population groups. In one example it was proposed that white, English and Afrikaans speaking patients tended to complain of feelings of sadness, insomnia and loss of appetite. Conversely, it was suggested that black, seSotho speaking patients expressed symptoms of mental illness in slightly different ways, such as complaining of "warm blood" and more physical ailments – making DSM diagnoses difficult. Furthermore, it was suggested that the different presentations of mental illness lead sufferers to seek care from traditional healers, who were completely absent in the collaboration network of the study. Co-morbidity was cited as a major distraction in diagnosing psychosis, in that psychosis was perceived as a very common symptom of pneumonia, meningitis and HIV. A senior psychiatrist alleged that trauma doctors often refer patients presenting with psychosis directly to the psychiatry unit without further examination, leading to serious conditions such as tuberculosis and HIV being missed. Some were highly sceptical of any form of recovery outside the medical sphere, noting that NGOs should "take the patient when you need and bring it back, because psychiatric will remain psychiatric until they die. That doesn't change" (PN_DH2).

Both public and private participants suggested that many mental health service providers did not have an adequate understanding and appreciation for the complexity of mental health care. Participants rarely distinguished different types or classifications of mental illness. Differentiations that were made largely related to manageability and functioning of patients. Some participants used terms such as 'mental disability', 'mental retardation', 'mental illness', and 'psychotic' interchangeably. People living with mental illness were pejoratively referred to as "mentals", "psychiatrics", and schizophrenics". Often, little or no distinction was made between mental illness and mental disability, a conflation that assumed lower cognitive ability. Serious mental disorders such as bipolar disorder and schizophrenia dominated discussions on mental illness, and narratives related to psychosis, dangerousness, risk and confinement emerged. Accounts unfolded underwritten by the need for police intervention in cases where patients became "uncontrollable" and "dangerous", especially in the absence of adequate medical intervention. Most participants relied heavily on police assistance when confronted with people suffering from psychosis. Some questioned the suitability (as well as the willingness) of the police to transport people suffering from psychosis. A lack of police training in managing psychosis was a concern, the impetus placed on subduing the person in question by any means. This idea was closely related to approaches to mental illness in comparison with other health concerns:

> *If you get a heart attack they call an ambulance, then the ambulance arrives and he will take you to the hospital. If a psychiatric guy is difficult, then who do they call? The police.*
>
> (CP_TH)

Though beyond the scope of this study, a few participants offered insight into the debilitating consequences of mental illness and the circumstances PWMI find themselves in. Stigma towards PWMI was often discussed: "The community does not view them as normal. So they are giving them names" (PN_DH1). Furthermore, it was suggested that PWMI had a slim chance to gain access to an open labour market. People whose condition debilitate them to the extent that they cannot access the labour market, are vitally dependent on a monthly disability grants paid to them by the DoSD via the South Africa Social Security Agency. In order to access this grant, they require assistance from a social worker and a physician. Within the contexts of abject poverty, many families become dependent on a grantee's disability stipend. Given the lack of public funding for mental health and social care, many NGOs providing housing and treatment adherence to their tenants used a proportion of clients' grant money to stay afloat.

A phenomenon materialised where PWMI became sources of capital for NGOs, an occurrence that – given the mentioned lack of regulatory oversight over NGOs – created spaces for incentives for people rather than for their care. This narrative emerged particularly in discussions on relationships between public and non-state service partners. One participant remarked that the state is similar to someone owning a Kentucky Fried Chicken franchise, but "…if you all take away his customer, he's got nothing. So those customers [NGOs] need him [PWMI], and the same with the state" (CC_NGO3). Subtle struggles emerged between public and private participants in terms of ownership of PWMI, exemplified by a PHC nurse complaining that collaborating NGO's boundaries of client retention:

> *Last time he even told sister on the phone that I'm even doing you people a favour for keeping these people here. He's doing us a favour? I don't know how. Because he's the one who's keeping the people*
>
> (PN_PHCC3)

Mental health stewardship

Mental health financing structures

Public mental health care were funded in two main ways. Facilities that provided mental health care in the public sphere received their funding from the DoH, while NGO services and disability grants were governed by the DoSD. The capacity of the state, especially DoSD, to provide funding was called in question, with one participant remarking, "Social Development is obviously non-existent or non-functional" (CP_PHCC4). However, in the context of splintered approaches to mental health as a programme and the lack of provincial policy direction, confusion emerged from some NGOs in terms of under which sectoral governance structures operate.

Adding to confusion was the muddling of the roles of social workers employed by the DoH vis-à-vis social workers employed by the DoSD. DoH social workers were confined to hospital and clinic settings, while DoSD social workers were allowed into community settings. Participants stated that DoH is involved in screening for mental illness, though some were unsure to which extent DoSD funded NGOs provided housing and treatment adherence to PWMI. Funding seemed to be closely tied to the physical nature of disability. One NGO commented that they only started to engage with DoH after self-harm became a problem for clients suffering from addiction. The link between the visible infirmities and funding were further illustrated by the following narrative:

> *But, it is very difficult to get grants for these poor people, because it isn't a physical disability that one can see. One cannot see that his arm is off or that he is blind or whatever. So they have to provide ten times the proof before they are willing to give these poor people a disability grant.*
>
> (CC_NGO2)

State funding for mental health focused on secondary and tertiary care, where most of mental health professionals were concentrated, which detracted funding from community mental health and PHC. PWMI, who have medical insurance, largely accessed services from a for-profit, private psychiatric hospital. The hospital was established in the context of an expanding private health care sector that did not include psychiatric services. As suggested by one participant, the real "money spinner" in general hospitals are theatre costs associated with surgery, while psychiatry costs are reduced to beds (where physicians are private contractors in this agreement) (CC_NGO8). This laid the foundation for a flourishing private psychiatric sector. Contributing to the previously mentioned theme of patients-as-capital, dissatisfaction was expressed by both public and private participants towards the management of medically insured patients by the private for-profit hospital, illustrated as:

> *What we see is that they [the private for-profit psychiatric hospital] refer guys to us after exhausting their funds. So they keep the guy there, deplete his funds and then there's some sort of crisis and then they say, go to [non-profit NGO], they'll do it for free as a state patient. It's a little hard to swallow.*
>
> (CC_NGO5)

Prioritisation

The aforementioned court case that the NGO coalition brought against the state resulted in the court ordering clear-cut prioritisation of welfare programme spending. In this vein, the state were tasked with developing a priority list for funding NGO activities, with mental health care and substance abuse rehabilitation activities being shifted significantly down the priority list. Apart from this formal directive, it was also remarked that for DOSD mental health was "*not generally a passion – their focus is children*" (SW_TH). NGOs that are subsidised by the DoSD to provide housing to those in need were identified as more likely to receive funding if their tenants are physically disabled – they mentioned "invisibility" of mental illness as a barrier to prioritisation. This prioritisation was also linked to global health funding priorities. Some NGOs mentioned that they had to frame their mental health work in terms of overlap with HIV and tuberculosis programmes in order to access funding. They mentioned that "mental health drinks out of a large pot, from which many others drink" (CP_PHCC4), and that it "suckles on the back teat [getting the short end of the stick] when it comes to funding and support" (CC_NGO2). A perception emerged that the state is "tightening the screws in order to push guys who get funding out of the system, because funds are depleting" (CC_NGO7).

Despite singular instances of participants who suggested that provincial support for mental health was exemplary, it was asserted that the state does not take mental health programs seriously. Some noted that the provincial government made chimerical promises that do not translate any national programmatic directives into tangible outcomes, including fostering non-state collaboration. Further, it was noted that mental health is completely absent from current health reforms such as National Health Insurance and the overhaul of PHC systems. There was a discussion on integrating mental health into PHC clinics, in accordance with national policy guidelines. The current absence of mental health in PHC settings was perceived as a feature of an "archaic health system". The absence of a mental health directorate until 2013 hampered the delivery of mental health care in PHC settings, though the nature of integration was somewhat misunderstood, and "integration" was reduced to screening for mental illness in PHC settings. In addition, the validity of the mental health screening tool was called into question, and only two of the seven questions were perceived to have any relevance, namely "Have you ever felt like killing yourself?", and "Do you often feel angry or worried?" One participant suggested that the screening tool was developed in haste only after a directive from top managers that mental health should receive more attention. Consequently, it was remarked that mental health "is dying a slow death" (PN_PHCC1). It was noted that existing state responses to mental illness as a public health programme were largely reactive, and not preventative as underlined in policy: "I think that patients are only helped once they really end up on the streets" (SW_TH).

Strategic leadership

Senior professionals noted that their inputs in policy processes and strategic decisions are routinely ignored, with one participant remarking that mental health policy is national-driven. This observation was backed by another participant, who did not see the necessity of translating national policies into provincial contexts, framing the development of contextual provincial policy as redundant. Occasional friction sometimes emerged between national and provincial spheres of governance:

> *Regarding welfare, there is really an unhealthy conflict between the national departments and the provincial departments. The national department wants more power, which is good and bad, while the provincial guys also cling to their power because they say they want their own thing.*
>
> (CC_NGO4)

An urgency regarding the need for competent, "dynamic expert leaders" emerged. This was not directed only to provincial-level leadership, but also to facility management. Over-bureaucratic structures and poor management resulted in the little funding assigned to mental health being mismanaged, frustrating public mental health professionals doing community outreach. A participant indicated that in one instance, after funds allocated to psychiatric community outreach work was depleted, the DoH assigned the team a helicopter (that was budgeted for in another programme but not appropriately used). A senior psychiatrist remarked "Yes, it was very nice for us, but my wife said that it was a [expletive] absurdity, absurdity. It is ridiculous, yes" (P_PHCC4). The fragmentation and disjuncture of mental health care delivery as a public health programme, especially between DoH and DoSD, did not only emerge in collaborative relationships, but was also as a feature of provincial state leadership. The political nature of public appointments was questioned, highlighted by the sentiment that the state "appoints teachers as hospital administrators" (CP_TH). One participant summed this sentiment up by alluding to Plato: "Expertise should be able to manage expertise, because if expertise does not administer expertise, it's something else" (CP_PHCC4).

Information and monitoring system

Using and generating information is a crucial aspect of stewardship, and many gaps emerged. A senior public official noted that policy objectives should be measured from a national perspective, suggesting that "by 2020 somebody has to review to check whether you actually achieved what you wanted to achieve" (MHCC). In line with the mentioned structural fragmentation, a fractured information system emerged, each NGO with its own paper-based forms, and public facilities with no mental health register, and minimal indicators, without any suggestion that this information is shared or used for strategic decision-making. Most information of patients suffering from mental illness were captured in paper-based files, that often were lost, in which case nurses had to engage with the patient by memory. In many cases, patients who accessed on-going care and stopped their treatment for more than a year had their case histories disposed of by the hospital – this necessitated PHC-level staff to re-create patient records in order to admit the patient to secondary levels of care. Further, the fractured information system made referrals challenging, especially in referral between public and non-state providers, where the responsibility often shifted to the patient:

> *So as soon as this person walks out of here, we don't know. Because they never bring back, like even our patients themselves never bring it back to us and say: "I went there and this is what happened". So we're not sure what happens at the end.*
>
> (PN_PHCC3)

Resistance

Instances of resistance to existing mental health care public governance emerged. Some participants believed that to have their interests satisfied they had to subvert traditional government hierarchies. Following the official lines of communication in public departments rarely led to desired outcomes, and more than one participant mentioned the importance of having direct access to the politically elected (and powerful) departmental head. A mental health nurse employed by a public hospital had to visit NGOs after work hours in order to circumvent managerial policy that prohibits employees from working outside the public sphere. Some public participants worked with private participants to circumvent referral steps in order to expedite access to specialist care for PWMI. Normally, someone with mental illness is required to a) present to a PHC clinic for screening (which occurs only once a month in some of the more rural clinics), b) after which referral to a district or regional hospital occurs (where there is a paucity of psychiatrists, who are sanctioned to provide clinical diagnosis and treatment), and c) after which referral to a specialist psychiatric hospital and psychiatric assistance can occur. Public health workers assist non-state organisations to obtain an order for involuntary admission to the psychiatric hospital according to the Mental Health Act (even if it is not strictly necessary) that provides PLWMI access more swiftly than traditional routes.

The severity of mental illness of patients was sometimes inflated in order to secure a disability grant, and it was highlighted that "depression does not qualify", and that psychotic features are stressed towards facilitating disability grant access. In this way, schizophrenia and bipolar disorder are more desirable as a diagnosis (PN_PHCC1). Some of the NGOs claimed that they had to frame their activities in certain ways in order to be successful in gaining access to state funding – this included framing mental health as a HIV-related challenge, and diminishing its faith-based approach to appear more secular. One NGO made it clear that they refuse to work with the DoSD, because of the overly bureaucratic and stringent nature of assessing NGOs for state subsidy. Some were adamant that mental health care should not be unified, claiming that "the bottom line is, the state should care for who it is supposed to care for, and the private [sector] should care for the private" (CC_NGO8).

Discussion

Mental health and its governance were found to be highly fragmented – most strikingly in terms of public and non-state service providers, biomedical and social approaches to care, and disjuncture between the DoH and DoSD. The schism between public and non-state spheres was particularly striking, and the relation between the two service domains suggested resource-based influences, supporting previous indications that the resource-based power of NGOs significantly influence their relations with public government (van Pletzen et al. 2014). These dichotomies block optimal collaboration and cooperation, and include key barriers to integrated care: professional domain conflicts; power relationships between services and professionals; distrust; vertical relationships with government; differences in expertise, organisational culture and service delivery approaches; bureaucratic structures; unclear roles; and funding mechanisms (Browne et al. 2004; Glendinning 2003; Kodner & Spreeuwenberg 2002; Wihlman, Lundborg, Axelsson, & Holmström 2008).

Several themes related to public stewardship of mental health care emerged. Broadly, stewardship involves the governance of health system rules, ensuring equity among health providers and among health providers and patients, and setting providing strategic leadership for the health system as a whole (Murray & Frenk 2000). Strong leadership is a particularly strong mechanism in health system strengthening (Gilson 2007), and along with cross-sectoral approaches to health, it forms a protective barrier around public health in the context of competing interests (Frenk & Moon 2013). Indeed, a key feature of stewardship is the building of supportive coalitions towards policy-specific outcomes (Rispel & Setswei 2007; World Health Organization 2000). Our findings particularly illuminate previous suggestions of poor information systems and monitoring of mental health in LMICs (Hanlon et al. 2014), and affirms that provincial government managers hold significant power over programme funding and information (Lehmann & Gilson 2013). Strategic leadership was also cast in a negative light, a weakness that becomes more pressing against the background of broad and ambitious health system reforms such as the re-engineering of PHC and the introduction of a national health insurance scheme, as well as the identified need for structural and organisational reorientation towards improved cooperation (Gilson & Daire 2011).

Having gained traction from its earlier beginnings, stewardship has been billed as one of the cornerstones of health system improvement, and "at its best, could provide an organizing principle for power in society transcending economics to base itself on the common interest" (Saltman & Ferroussier-Davis 2000, 735). Nevertheless, power is a nebulous concept, and framing its dynamics under the guise of serving interests is limiting – many other forms of power are at play (Deleuze 2004). In our findings public and formal health system hierarchies emerged as forms of power that guided the referral and collaborative behaviour of the mental health service network. Hierarchies and budgetary controls as forms of power – not subsisting in any individual or specific institution (Foucault 1980) – have been suggested elsewhere to be a feature of local health care provision in South Africa (Lehmann & Gilson 2013).

Further, it seems prudent to ask whose interests are being served within the stewardship and governance dynamic, and how policy subjects are problematized (Bacchi 2010). In this vein, we build on a narrative of competing public health priorities as a stark reality faced by PWMI in LMICs (Hanlon et al. 2014). The setting of public health priorities seemed to be strongly rooted in terms of certain types of differential value. Programmes such as HIV and tuberculosis were deemed more important than mental health; physical disability was deemed more pressing than mental disability; and children and the elderly attracted more funding than PWMI. The worst example of this type of prioritisation was illustrated in the Life Esidimeni crisis, where following the financial de-prioritisation of severe mental illness in a South African province led to 94 preventable deaths of deinstitutionalised patients suffering from severe mental conditions (Makgoba 2017). It is a strategy employed by a state with neoliberal tendencies, where specific populations are stratified and codified, often to their disadvantage (Wacquant 2009a, 2009b).

Mental health care is couched in the governance sphere of the DoH, but the position of NGOs under the governance sphere of the DoSD elevates the importance of multi-sectoral coordination. Such ideals are however hampered by structural divisions, separate policy and administrative spheres, complex and dissimilar funding structures, and distinctive professional backgrounds (Mur-Veeman et al. 2008; Nicaise et al. 2013). Further, contestations among provincial programme managers often echo through to service delivery levels (Lehmann & Gilson 2013), a phenomenon that emerged in our study. The lack of integration between biomedical-oriented and socially-oriented mental health care – a persisting challenge emphasised before (Petersen 2000) – is particularly salient due to the nature of mental illness, which generally falls at the interface of biomedical health and social services (Rummery 2009).

Professional boundaries are in line with different understanding of and approaches to the classification, causes and treatment of mental illness, that have contributed to disjointed mental health care systems (Plagerson 2015). A bridge in this sense seemed to be the social work profession, who were highlighted to be particularly important referral agents, both to public and non-state service providers. Collaborations that involve significant social work engagement can elevate the voice of patients, as well as increase community organisation improvements and social capital (Hultberg, Lonnroth, & Allebeck 2005; Postle & Beresford 2007; Rummery 2009). The importance of social work here is not only rooted in social workers' professional positions, but also an indication of deeper, more subtle forms of power in collaborative care (Janse van Rensburg et al. 2016). As suggested by Nikolas Rose (Carvalho 2015), "social work is a kind of technology", involving a specific type of training and authority. Social workers certainly are not alone in this power dynamic, and the mental health professions each play a role in the management of people rendered subjects of state intervention.

In this way, the police (Foucault 1980), psychiatric nurses (Holmes & Gastaldo 2002), psychologists (Binkley 2011), and psychiatrists (Rose 1996b) all play a part in the governmentality of mental illness. To these idiosyncrasies of advanced liberalism and late capitalism (Carvalho 2015) we can further add the commodification of PWMI that emerged in the findings. The state fosters legitimacy by claiming to provide for the well-being of the population, driven by an instrumental economic rationality of costs and benefits (Chatterjee 2004). Under these conditions, PLWMI – who have little chance of entering and remaining in the labour market – personifies Homo Sacer, the cast out, where "bare life" becomes the authentic subject of politics (Agamben 1998). They essentially exist under a "spectre of uselessness", a challenge to the state provision of welfare benefits (Sennett 2006). The state provides the infrastructure that fosters supportive conditions for the working of quasi-markets (Carvalho 2015), and the framing of PWMI as "useless" in modern society transforms them into objects of economic rationalities. These claims are demonstrated in our findings, in terms of PWMI getting caught up in a complex network where there are financial and information flows between public departments, between public and non-state service providers, and in interactions with for-profit psychiatric services.

Thus far, many different facets of power have been unearthed. Yet, "where there is power, there is resistance" (Foucault 1980, 95), and resistance is a central feature of power dynamics involving health care providers and government intervention (Doolin 2004). Within collaborative contexts, resistance often emerges in relation to power distribution and decision-making structures (Nilsen, Dugstad, Eide, Gullslett, & Eide 2016). In our findings, resistance emerged in several forms: resistance against funding structures (framing applications for welfare grants in certain ways); resistance against hierarchical power structures (bypassing referral lines in order to gain access to specialist mental health professionals); and resistance against the public and non-state divide (public mental health care professionals who visit NGOs in order provide care). The NGO that refused to engage with government funding structures is reminiscent of a form of passive resistance, a withdrawal from formal health system interfaces (Lehmann & Gilson 2013). These forms of resistance – while closely intertwined in the power dynamics within which it operates (Foucault 1980), can be interpreted as strategies that resist smooth and "complete malleability in the idealised schemes of a programmatic logic" (Miller & Rose 2008)71.

Finally, the limitations of our theoretical framework (Purdy 2012) should be assessed. While a theoretical framework provides the researcher with "a map for combining the what with the why to gain a multidimensional understanding" of the phenomenon under focus (Evans, Coon, & Ume 2011), no framework is without critique. In our study, we were confronted by a common problem in research, namely discrepancies between neatly delineated theoretical constructs and the messy reality of collaboration and local governance. The framework does not adequately encapsulate the informal, non-descript forms of contact between collaborators that emerged in our study, and we had to adjust accordingly. Further, the framework did not pay sufficient attention to the surrounding contexts of collaborative relationships, of which there are considerations. Governance and collaborative dynamics are nested in wider systems (Emerson, Nabatchi, & Balogh 2012), and our inductive amendment of public stewardship is one example of such a consideration. Nevertheless, use of the framework provided a necessary degree of robustness to the study, and offers the flexibility required for use in different contexts.

Conclusion

Mental illness truly represents a "wicked problem" in health policy (Hannigan & Coffey 2011), as its nature necessitates that it "axiomatically transcends a diverse range of professional and organizational boundaries and often at multiple levels" (Hunter & Perkins 2012, 45). Non-state mental health service providers are a real and important component of national health systems in LMICs, and close engagement between public and non-state actors is a key consideration towards achieving universal health coverage (Alliance for Health Policy and Systems Research 2015). The significance of this chapter is rooted in its empirical illustration of local mental health service governance dynamics in a South African context. Importantly, the complexities and different facets of power dynamics that underwrite attempts towards integrated mental health care are showcased, adding to growing literature on the social mechanisms that influence collaboration. The study confirms and expands on previous studies of the crucial role of health system governance in South African settings (Hanlon et al. 2017; Inge Petersen et al. 2017a; Scott et al. 2014), and, importantly, illuminates the role of power in integration and fragmentation of mental health services (Janse van Rensburg et al. 2016). Nowhere has power emerged more vividly in mental health care than in the Life Esidimeni case, the subject of the next chapter.

Note

1 This chapter has been previously published in the *International Journal of Health Planning and Management*.

6 When systems fail

Life Esidimeni and the meaning of justice

Introduction

Thus far we have discussed the boundaries of South Africa's post-apartheid mental health system, with specific reference to people with severe mental and neurological conditions, who do not have the financial support to access private for-profit care. We have drawn the contours of care along the line of state, for-profit private care, and non-profit CSOs, who interact with each other in various (largely uncoordinated) ways, with different motivations. We have touched on events that have challenged these relations, but none has had such a significant impact on the public discourse about how we as a society care for the vulnerable than the Life Esidimeni crisis. The many, many opinions levied about this tragedy tended to follow a similar theme: corrupt, incompetent politicians, with malicious intent, forcibly moved a group of vulnerable people to CSOs, portrayed as places of misery and death. The Ombud's report, which would become a key reference during the saga, used the comparison to concentration camps to drive this point home (Makgoba 2017). Commenting on the Life Esidimeni crisis, as well as on the SASSA crisis, the editor for the South African Medical Journal remarked that

> The "canary in the coal mine" analogy is apt. We can no longer close our eyes to the corruption and wilful neglect of our public services, and indeed our people, by a government that is increasingly desperate to hold on to power, and through it access to the public purse. The imminent crisis around the distribution of social grants on 1 April this year is another case in point. If this distribution fails, lack of these grants will cause massive hardship, and quite possibly illness and death, for yet another group of voiceless and vulnerable people.
>
> (Farham 2017, 277)

These considerations are hard to contest. Nevertheless, by focusing on the actions of agents (which can mean people, organisations or political parties), we lose sight of the much more persisting effects of structure. The Ombud who penned the influential report, Malegapuru Makgoba, highlighted three lessons that we should learn from the crisis: (1) to re-think our bioethics, which is still rooted in apartheid and colonial thinking; (2) we should move beyond denial of faults and confront problems head-on; and (3) we should address political interference in independent bodies (NGO Pulse 2018). In the wake of collective sense-making of the event, very little reflection emerged on the more systemic, deeper nuances that underwrite how decisions and priorities are made. Wendy Brown remarked that political scandals are often "framed as a matter of miscalculation or political manoeuvring rather than by right and wrong, truth or falsehood, institutional propriety or impropriety", thereby concealing the evisceration of democratic principles and, more importantly, democratic morality (Brown 2003).

In this vein, the purpose of this Chapter is to interrogate the structural effects of South Africa's public socioeconomic sphere on the ways in which people with severe mental illness are governed, using the Life Esidimeni crisis as an illustrative example. It ultimately seeks to explore the achievement of justice in the wake of the event, and what justice might mean for people with severe mental and neurological conditions more broadly.

The Life Esidimeni crisis: A brief timeline

Unfolding of events

The timeline of the Life Esidimeni tragedy is well-described. During its unfolding, several media platforms monitored the events; public attention was significantly ramped up during the release of the Ombud Report, and the event became global once the public arbitration process was set in motion. The last time so much attention was paid to a human rights issue in South Africa, was two decades before during the Truth and Reconciliation (TRC) hearings. Despite the general familiarity of the crisis, it is prudent to provide a short timeline that we can draw from to identify salient analytical slices that can help expose the fundamental undercurrent that ultimately established a context within which it would become possible to create so much devastation. A rudimentary timeline is presented in Figure 6.1.

The Life Esidimeni tragedy was formally put into motion in a budget speech on 19 June 2019, when GDoH MEC Qedani Mahlangu announced

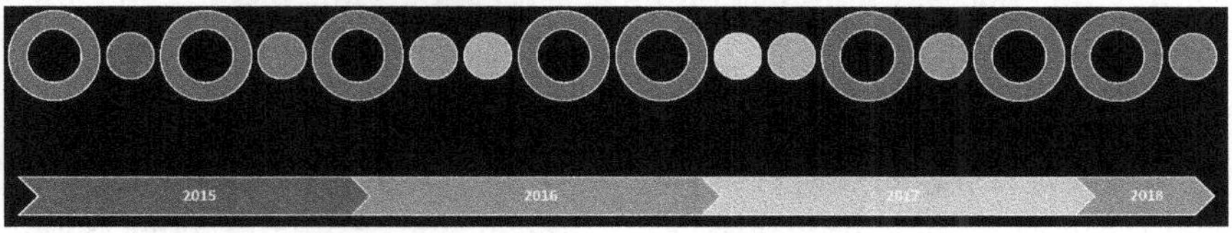

Figure 6.1 A timeline of the Life Esidimeni tragedy.

that the contractual relationship between the province and Life Health care would not be renewed (Mahlangu 2015a). Two reasons were provided. First, it was argued that this decision falls in line with requirements of Chapter Two of the Mental Health Care Act (17 of 2002): "Persons providing care, treatment and rehabilitation services must provide such services in a manner that facilitates community care of mental health care users" (Subsection Six) (South African Government 2002). Second, the GDoH argued that the amount of $24 million being spent on 2 378 patients during the 2014/2015 financial year was unaffordable, and that those funds would be reprioritised elsewhere (Mahlangu 2015b). The announcement of the Marathon plans came at the back end of a particularly challenging fiscal year for the GDoH. During 2014/2015, care for 2,378 patients at Life Esidimeni cost the GDoH 1% of its R31.5 billion budget (around R323.7 million), and the plan was initially to reduce the number of Life Esidimeni beneficiaries slowly up until 2020. However, the GDoH had well-known financial woes, and its 2014/2015 audit report flagged an overspending of R72 million (Comrie 2016). The purported financial pressure was a key motivating factor presented by the GDoH to legitimise the Gauteng Mental Health Marathon Project.

The decision to end the contract, along with the purported reasons behind it, opened up a discursive space which allowed an unveiling of the true nature of how we as a society respond to severe mental and neurological conditions – particularly among the poor. In time, it became clear that the decision to deinstitutionalise the Life Esidimeni victims in this particular way was not simply made by an apparently corrupt and/or incompetent individual (if you followed media reports), but was firmly embedded in complex political, historical and socioeconomic structures. The plan to move people with severe mental and neurological conditions from the care of Life Esidimeni to CSOs was part of the Gauteng Mental Health Marathon Project, an initiative aimed to fast-track deinstitutionalisation and community-based care. Following the unveiling of the Gauteng Mental Health Marathon Project plans and timelines, the South African Society for Psychiatrists (SASOP) and the South African Depression and Anxiety Group (SADAG) had fierce engagement with the GDoH to try and delay the initiation of the planned move. SASOP, as the official body of the psychiatry profession in SA, had a particularly high stake in the planned move. Afterall, psychiatry is the custodian of professional knowledge in the clinical management of severe mental conditions. As a medical speciality, psychiatry is firmly rooted in hard historical lessons learnt during the deinstitutionalisation debacle in the United States and other countries during the 1970s and 1980s.[1] Speaking from these painful histories, SASOP and SADAG underlined the critical need for an adequate community safety net prior to any discharge of patients. After the GDoH decided to go ahead despite these concerns, a series of stakeholder meetings were held to delay the move. Again, the main concern from mental health stakeholders were South Africa's critical lack of a coordinated, resourced community mental health system. This deficiency has been repeatedly highlighted (Bernard Janse van Rensburg 2011; Krüger & Lewis 2011; Moosa & Jeenah 2008). In fact, the GDoH were clamping down on illegal (meaning, unregistered) "halfway houses" just a year before, closing down eight in 2014. Funding for the opening and support of such facilities were however not forthcoming (Mkhwanazi 2015). It should also be added here that the specific population we are discussing – namely people with severe mental and neurological conditions *and* who are socioeconomically disadvantaged – tend to suffer the brunt of societal challenges. David Rochefort (1997, 236) noted that "The severely mentally ill are multiply disadvantaged by poverty, disability, lack of housing and employment opportunities and persistent social stigma", requiring a public mental health care system that abolishes discriminating structures and repairs "the social 'safety net' to make it truly comprehensive and reliable". This is far from a ground-breaking revelation, and it is assumed that this is an established truth in public health. Despite clear, merited warnings, the GDoH argued that financial constraints pushed them to a point where "the rehabilitation and discharge of mental health care users to either their homes or NGOs, earlier than was the practice before, is now an unavoidable priority of the department", and that they were merely following the national policy directive that people need to be cared for in the least restrictive environment possible. This claim was undercut by a GDoH spokesperson that said that the profiles of patients were not considered, but rather the costs (Comrie 2016). SADAG added their voice to a growing and urgent pushback to the plans.

As in the NAWONGO case, there was a coordinated, collective, court-based challenge to the state's attempt to initiate the Marathon plans. In a historic move, Section 27, supported by SASOP and other mental health stakeholder organisations, took the GDoH to the South Gauteng High Court to oppose (what was argued to be) the unilateral decision to proceed with the deinstitutionalisation plans. The Court recommended that the parties settle out of court by January 2016; but when this deadline elapsed, GDoH took the opportunity to proceed. An urgent interdict application to the Court was dismissed after the GDoH managed to convince the judge that they still adhered to the original agreement. Ultimately though, a sizeable collection of professional and non-governmental organisations formally opposed the GDoH's plans, including SASOP, SADAG, the South African Medical Association (SAMA), the Psychological Society of South Africa (PsySSA), Rural Rehab South Africa, People's Health Movement SA, the Treatment Action Campaign (TAC), the Public Health Association of SA's Mental Health Special Interest Group, SAMA's Junior Doctors Association of SA (JUDASA), and Section 27 (for a discussion on non-organisational pushback during this time, see Janse van Rensburg 2017).

Despite attempted blocks from the professional mental health community, firmly embedded in relative certainty about what happens when deinstitutionalisation without adequate community support takes place, the GDoH pushed the move through. The initial plan was to send patients (deemed functional enough) home to their families, while 526 of the more severe cases were to be sent to Weskoppies and Sterkfontein psychiatric hospitals, institutions already buckling under psychiatric backlogs (to some extent, due to the lack of community-based mental health care) (Comrie 2016). The contract was formally ended on 31 March 2016, which was extended until 30 June 2016 to accommodate the transfer. From 1 April to 30 June 2016 alone, 1,371 patients were discharged, at a rate of 457 patients per month compared to 13.3 patients per month the previous year. The exponential speed and rushed nature of the transfer became a central point of critique – subsequent opinions put the desired time required for such a transition at 5 years minimum (Makgoba 2017). Patients were ultimately transferred to 27 CSOs, none of whom were licenced by the DoH or DoSD. Prior to the transfer, various CSOs were invited to submit proposals to receive contracts, some applied for licences, some underwent pre-placement audits – no pilot placements were done. What is clear though, is that most of the CSOs had little to no experience in caring for people with severe mental and neurological conditions, and were woefully inappropriate for the task at hand. Initial agreements with CSOs were changed later, when numbers of transferred users were numbers were increased, and some received men instead of women (or vice versa). Some CSOs specialised in other programmes, for instance taking care of orphaned children, or promoting female empowerment. Simply put, the CSOs were

> mysteriously and poorly selected, poorly prepared, "not ready", their staff was not trained, not qualified and was unable to distinguish between the highly specialized non-stop professional care requirements of 'assisted' Mental Health Care User (MCHU) from LE and a business opportunity; there were often mismatches between MCHU functionality with NGO fitness for purpose.
>
> (Makgoba 2017, 2)

Then, there was the element of human dignity – patients were received via trucks, open bakkies, and in a generally uncoordinated manner; in states of dishevelment, some without shoes and with torn clothes, unwashed. The following section refers:

> Some "without wheel chairs but tied with bed sheets" to support them; some NGOs rocked up at LE in open "bakkies" to fetch MCHUs while others chose MCHUs like an "auction cattle market" despite pre-selection by the GDMH staff; some MCHUs were shuttled around several NGOs; during transfer and after deaths several relatives of patients were still not notified or communicated to timeously; some are still looking for relatives; these conducts were most negligent and reckless and showed a total lack of respect for human dignity, care and human life.
>
> (Makgoba 2017, 2)

Some were moved to CSOs they were not notified of, or moved and removed several times. In terms of clinical needs, the chronic medication prescription refill cycles were not communicated to CSOs, posing substantial harm to continuity of psychopharmaceutical care. Physical comorbidities were ignored, to the degree that conditions such as skin sores and hypertension were aggravated in the absence of appropriate care. Astonishingly, this happened without informing the families, and when the deaths started emerging, chaos ensued.

Family members of the transferred, having little success locating their loved ones through official state channels, turned to the media for help. Stories gained traction about missing and dead people, and pressure started to mount on the GDoH to provide answers. By August 2016 Christine Nxumalo, sister of one of the victims who died at a CSO, wrote a public letter to the DoH to demand answers, adding a human dimension to the pressure. On 13 September 2016, the MEC announced that 36 patients had died during the transfer process, which unleashed a flood of condemnation – two days later, health minister Dr Aaron Motsoaledi requested an official enquiry from the OHSC. This was to be the first major task for the newly-appointed Ombud, Prof Malegapuru Makgoba, and he initiated a comprehensive investigation.

The Ombud Report

The 56-page report was the result of analyses of clinical and other patient-level records by an eight-person expert panel; the CSOs involved were investigated by means of on-site visits, inspections and interviews by two OHSC inspectors; the investigation team reviewed popular media coverage, documents, and case presentations with affidavits from civil society group Section 27, and worked with Statistics South Africa to analyse mortality; and the Ombud interviewed 73 individuals under oath or affirmation. The findings of the investigation entail wide-spread condemnation of the Life Esidimeni transfer process, as well as the mental health system as a whole. The report concluded that not 36 people, but more than 94 died during the transfer process (Makgoba 2017). The release of the report was delayed by the MEC needing to give input, but ultimately, it was released on 1 February 2017 – the MEC resigned on the same day. The Ombud Report became *the* source of reference for the Life Esidimeni saga, and a slew of newspaper articles, opinion pieces and cartoons flooded the public sphere. The MEC was particularly derided, and many commentators saw this as a symptom of an increasingly corrupt and inefficient state under the leadership of Zuma's ANC. An almost universal agreement emerged that the Life Esidimeni events was an abuse of basic human rights. The report is a complete indictment of the GDoH, and thoroughly debunked their purported reasons for initiating the Gauteng Mental Health Marathon Project. It showed that the absence of community mental health care was well-known and that the GDoH repeatedly ignored the many calls from prominent stakeholders to cease the operation. Importantly, the Report showed that the assertions by MEC Mahlangu that her department could not afford the costs of US$22.50 per patient per day at Life Esidimeni, when this rate was substantially lower than market rate. For instance, costs per patient per day at state-funded Weskoppies, Sterkfontein Cullinan Care and Rehabilitation Centre hospitals were calculated at US$137.82, US$97.45 and US$104.47, respectively (Makgoba 2017).

Recommendations from the Report involved disciplinary proceedings against key GDoH officials; legal proceedings taken against CSOs involved in preventable deaths; a review of the regulatory position of CSOs involved in the Marathon Project; the National Minister of Health was instructed to immediately appoint a task team to review licencing regulations and procures involved in regulating CSOs, in line with various legal frameworks; a review and harmonisation of the National Health Act and the Mental Health Care Act to streamline different spheres of government and centralise certain functions to the national health minister. It is not certain to what degree these tasks have been completed to date.

Nonetheless, one of the key recommendations – that the national health minister should request the South African Human Rights Council (SAHRC) to undertake a systemic review of mental health human rights compliance and violations across provinces – was taken up. A four-person panel, made up of SAHRC commissioners and a public mental health expert, conducted a comprehensive review of the state of the South African mental health system, from a human rights perspective. Written and oral submissions were made on record to the panel, by representatives of both government and non-government spheres: national and provincial departments of health; the DoSD; National Treasury; the Departments of Basic Education, Planning, Monitoring and Evaluation, Justice and Constitutional Development, Correctional Services, Human Settlements; South African Police Services; SAFMH; Ubuntu Centre; Rural Mental Health Campaign (RMHC); SASOP; the Deinstitutionalisation Task Team; and various key individuals and advocates in public mental health care. Key findings from this process are presented in Box 4, and mostly relate to a pressing need to implement national policy and legal guidelines. With respect to recommendations to specific provincial departments, deadlines were provided for the establishment of key mental health system structures, for instance the institution of district mental health teams, and intersectoral forums. None of the recommendations were surprising, or controversial – all spoke to well-known system deficits. Now it was up to provinces to fulfil their constitutional mandate and operationalise the ideals of the Mental Health Care Act and the National Mental Health Policy Framework and Strategic Plan. While this push was a necessary part of kick-starting reform, there remains a dire need for tools and strategies aimed to build technical expertise and leadership capacity for provincial and district management. It is here after all, where the different strands of service delivery need to be pulled together, coordinated, funded and monitored.

Box 6.1 Key findings from the National Hearing on the Status of Mental Health Care in South Africa (South African Human Rights Commission 2017)

1. The numerous human rights concerns that have been highlighted in this investigation can be said to arise out of a prolonged and systemic neglect of mental health at the level of policy implementation.
2. South Africa needs to make substantial progress on numerous fronts in order for the country to meet its obligations in terms of the Convention on the Rights of Persons with Disabilities (CRPD).
3. There is considerable under-investment in mental health by the South African government.
4. Comprehensive implementation of the NMHPF has not yet occurred.
5. Although the Mental Health Policy Framework and Strategic Plan (2013—2020) emphasizes the value of a primary health care approach in reducing the treatment gap, the provision of mental health services seems to focus on care in psychiatric hospitals.
6. The GMHMP has illustrated that deinstitutionalisation is a process that requires numerous interventions in various sectors to actualise the rights of people living with intellectual and psychosocial disabilities.
7. Many barriers to providing mental health services were highlighted and were particularly problematic in rural areas.
8. Participation of MHCUs in their treatment is a central component of a rights-based approach to mental health care.
9. Effective implementation of a rights-based approach to mental health requires an emphasis on the social determinants of mental health and well-being.
10. Services for children and adolescents are neglected.
11. The state of mental health services in the criminal justice, forensic and correctional systems in South Africa is particularly poor.
12. Broader conversations about law reform of instruments such as the MHCA and the Electoral Act are required.

Public arbitration and beyond

The massive media fallout from the report put the state under immense pressure to ensure that justice be served for the victims and this, much like during the TRC and Marikana hearings, resulted in a public arbitration process. On 9 October 2017, the process started, with open access to media, presided over by the much-respected Justice Dikgang Moseneke, calling on a wide range of testimonies. In his award statement, the judge opened by stating the following (laying the foundations on which the process would be built):

> This is a harrowing account of the death, torture and disappearance of utterly vulnerable mental health care users in the care of an admittedly delinquent provincial government. It is also a story of the searing and public anguish of the families of the affected mental health care users and of the collective shock and pain of many other caring people in our land and elsewhere in the world. These inhuman narratives were rehearsed before me, the Arbitrator, in arbitral proceedings I am about to describe.
> (Moseneke 2018)

The format of the event provided a much-needed degree of legitimacy, to show that the state was serious about addressing the social injustice of Life Esidimeni. A summary of the 44 days of hearings, as well as the full transcripts, can be accessed from the Bhekisisa Centre for Health Journalism (https://bhekisisa.org/article/2018-10-17-00-never-forget-download-the-full-life-esidimeni-tragedy-arbitration-transcripts/), but in short, the first three days, Malegapuru Makgoba and others provided a background to the events that unfolded, leading up to the death toll. Thereafter, there were testimonies speaking to a lack of coordination between national and provincial levels of government, as well as highlighting the disciplinary steps taken against state officials thus far. The days following these testimonies focused on describing the contexts of CSOs that accepted patients from Life Esidimeni, highlighting their inadequacies in caring for frail and vulnerable people with complex needs. This was followed by testimonies by family members describing their experiences in looking for and finding their loved ones, sharing the emotional toll the process took on them. The South African Police Service testified that their investigation was delayed by the GDoH's delay in supplying key documents, needing to revert to court action to obtain these documents. The chairperson of the Gauteng Mental Health Review Board testified that she did not know that she had the power to challenge the MEC's actions, and expressed a lack of understanding of the scope and duties of the Board. One of the CSOs admitted that they used their clients' disability grants to run their organisation, even still drawing funds from clients four months after being shut down by government. The nature of death of two of the victims were then described. On 10 November – Day 18 – the Health Ombud announced that the total death toll now stood at 144, with many remaining missing. A clinical psychologist testified that the Life Esidimeni actions were tantamount to torture, drawing parallels with concentration camps. Several CSOs then testified about their incapacity to deal with the influx of patients, with a lack of expertise, food and space being highlighted. There followed testimony of the internal processes of the GDoH that led to the transfer, with the Gauteng mental health services manager admitting that they knew about the lack of capacity of the CSOs. There was further discussion on the nature of deaths and the management of bodies post-mortem. A series of testimonies followed describing the lack of knowledge and consent from family members in terms of decisions made about the care of victims. The GDoH then testified that they proceeded with the transfer despite knowing that the required structures were not in place, and that the CSOs were not ready. A discussion also followed about the bioethics and professional code of conduct of the officials involved in the events.

Up until this point, ex-MEC Qedani Mahlangu – arguably the public face of the fiasco – had avoided participating in the arbitration process despite calls to attend. She had attended classes at the London School of Business and Finance, who subsequently suspended her following a public outcry. In January 2018 she took the stand, avoiding taking personal blame and denying having knowledge of the nature of the deaths. A psychiatrist testified that logically, the deaths could have been avoided, while a senior state finance official rubbished the claims that the aim of the Marathon Project was to save money. The premier of the province testified that he had no knowledge of the transfer from Life Esidimeni to CSOs. As the arbitration process drew to a close, the new Gauteng health MEC testified, as did Dr Aaron Motsoaledi, who described the Life Esidimeni events as "one of the most painful and horrible events in the history of post-apartheid South Africa", adding that "As minister of health, I wish to apologise unconditionally to the families and to all those who are still living. We have wronged them in a way unimaginable". Lawyers for both sides made final statements, after which the judge read his verdict. The judgement ordered the Gauteng provincial government to pay each of the 135 Life Esidimeni claimants R1 million each in Constitutional damages (the state was found to breach several sections of the Constitution, the National Health Act, and the Mental Health Care Act in contravention of the rights of the family members). Furthermore, the government was ordered to pay additional sums of R20,000 each for funeral costs, and R180,000 for psychological shock and trauma, bringing the total sum owed R1.2 million to each of the 135 families. Ultimately, the Gauteng Office of the Premier paid a total sum of R159.46-million in compensation.

The payments to families did not conclude the Life Esidimeni fiasco – to date, eight of the original transferees remain missing, almost five years after being moved. In February 2020, the Justice and Correctional Services Minister granted a request by the National Prosecuting Authority to conduct a joint hearing into the Life Esidimeni deaths, requesting the appointment of a judge to preside over the inquest in the Gauteng High Court. The end of the legal process is uncertain, though what is fairly clear, is that the health system lessons from Life Esidimeni have not been taken to heart. The focus on individual misdeeds cloaked the more serious health system issues that confound mental health care reform, especially the ideological and operational disengagement between the health and social sectors. Severe mental and neurological conditions were firmly ring-fenced in the health sphere, with little to no involvement from other sectors such as social development. The DoH has a hapless history of community-based interventions that require coordination beyond health facilities, and there is little doubt that community-based work requires a deep and real level of intersectoral working, with formal inclusion of civil society. The deep and persisting ruptures between the state and civil society, as was highlighted in the NAWONGO case, was not adequately acknowledged, nor any steps taken to resolve the fracture. During the beginning of the Life Esidimeni transfer, following the court interdict sought by civil society to slow the proceedings, the GDoH accused these organisations of being "dishonest" and acting with "selective morality" (Comrie 2016). The deep distrust followed throughout the transfer period and beyond. Apart from the demands made in the SAHRC report, little to no systematic evaluation data exist on progress in achieving the goals set out in the MHPF, apart from the obvious shortages in psychiatrists and psychologists. The myopic focus on the percentage of budgets spent on mental health, and citing the perpetually low mental health professionals to population ratio, has tended to blind the more fundamental challenges in South Africa's mental health system. If the Life Esidimeni tragedy taught us anything, it is that these shortcomings are lodged within structural dynamics that are yet to be fully explored.

A questionable justice

There have been many attempts to make sense of the Life Esidimeni events and to identify the central cause of the tragedy. Firstly, referring to the event as a tragedy is noteworthy. As Martha Nussbaum reminds us,

> Tragedy shows us that disasters do strike at the heart of human action: they don't just cause superficial discomfort, they impede mobility, planning, citizenship, ultimately life itself. On the other hand, when we see that such a disaster strikes a human being, it is then that we feel the sense of tragic compassion: for we don't want humanity to be wasted, or even callously pushed around.
>
> (Nussbaum 1998, np)

Lisi's (2015, 102) reading of Kierkegaard underlines the critical dilemma that confronts us in trying to make sense of Life Esidimeni as a tragedy, in that tragedy represents a "irreducible contradiction between two qualitatively distinct principles: substantial determinants and individual agency". The agency of the victims to prevent the dire outcomes that they had to experience was never seriously considered – their vulnerability due to their perceived incapacity to take care of themselves was after all the standard that allowed their institutionalisation in the first place. The focus rather fell firmly on the agency of individuals put in charge of their care. The ire of families and the broader public was particularly levelled at MEC Qedani Mahlangu, whose role as orchestrator of the event became a daily news story. This perceived role was aggravated by her reluctance to participate in the arbitration hearings, as well as her apparent lack of remorse (especially compared to Aaron Motsoaledi, who was visibly distraught during his testimony). Though she stepped down under immense public pressure, this was a bare minimum expectation. One of the families summed up their general sentiment: "I am not going to be happy until she is thrown in jail, her stepping down from the ANC is none of my business, that is just politics", (Maphanga 2018). To make matters worse, Mahlangu stood for and ultimately was elected into the Gauteng ANC provincial executive committee (PEC) in 2018, raising serious questions about the ANC's "moral core", and the meaning of justice in the aftermath of Life Esidimeni. It also echoed government accountability in the TRC and Marikana aftermath, strengthening the perception that state officials are not subject to the rule of law (Stanley 2001).

Penology teaches us that punishment takes can take on different colours, depending on contexts and the misconduct. We could incapacitate an individual, removing him or her from society, or we could prevent re-offending by rehabilitating the individual. In terms of the Life Esidimeni search for justice, the aim especially fell on restitution and retribution – the defendant had to be punished financially (R159.46 million paid by the GDoH), and the victims and society at broad needs to be given a feeling of avengement. This last dimension was clearly not achieved, even though there were multiple calls for disciplinary steps beyond financial damages. However, this particular approach to social justice is not entirely new or unique in South African contexts; this path was set by the TRC following the fall of apartheid, creating a frame against which many other social justice processes were subsequently pursued.

The TRC as a (unsatisfactory) blueprint for justice

The TRC was, at its core, an exercise in restorative justice through truth-seeking. It underlined a religious ideal, that reconciliation means that conflict should be addressing through mercy and forgiveness (Halpern & Weinstein 2004). By admitting, in an open and public space, politically driven crimes committed between 1960 and 1994, the TRC was empowered to provide individual amnesty. This was to be achieved through a dialogue between perpetrators, victims and community members. The idea was that this dialogue will uncover the truth about atrocities committed, through which victims' families could find a degree of solace and resolution, and perhaps start moving towards forgiveness and reconciliation (Androff 2009). The TRC was part of a broader peace-making deal between the apartheid government and Mandela's ANC, brokered to achieve stability following democratic transition. The process was lauded by many as being intrinsic to South Africa's peaceful transition, and gave rise to a series of other similar practices in countries seeking healing following political turmoil, especially in Rwanda, East Timor, and Sierra Leone. However, several voices have been critical towards its purported achieving a form of justice. While there undeniably was an ideal to achieve social justice through truth and reparations, this was not achieved in practice. At the root of this failure was a reticence from the new government to "rock the structural boat", an avoidance to challenge the status quo (Stanley 2001, 535). The public nature of the TRC did perhaps create a degree of symbolic justice, though in reality, "justice is most effective when it works in consort with other processes of social reconstruction and reflects the needs and wishes of those most affected by violence" (Weinstein & Stover 2004, 11). In this way, the goals of the TRC fell short, as it ultimately meant little in terms of people's daily lives (Clark 2012). By emphasising individual responsibility over institutional and structural accountability, certain culpable groups like the National Party could claim that crimes in their name were due to individual deviants rather than policy. Additionally, the general public, "ordinary" South African citizens, were absolved of blame, failing to recognise the "little perpetrator in us all" (Stanley 2001, 537). A central failure here was the nature of "truth" being pursued – the real degree to which people laid bare what happened will never truly be known, and, with this uncertainty, its potency in fostering justice was under suspicion. Additionally, and more pressingly, "Placed alongside continued inequality and discrimination, truth appears of little value" (Stanley 2001, 543). Poyner (2009), in analysing J. M. Coetzee's *Disgrace*, noted that the TRC uncovered truth at the cost of justice, that resources and capital have not been appropriately redistributed under the new democratic dispensation. Disgrace calls to question the nature of public versus private confession, where publicity warps the "true self". It also warns that neither individual nor institutional truths can be properly tested, and the authenticity required for justice to be achieved therefore falls short. Discourses of truth-telling, reparation and reconciliation are thus inherently political (Poyner 2009). Seeking justice in post-conflict settings requires that "truth must penetrate society to the extent that it helps to bring about fundamental changes in the way that people live their daily lives and relate to one another" – the extent to which truth is accepted in, and its ultimate effects within society need to be acknowledged, in other words, its role in shaping people's daily lives (Clark 2012, 191).

The spirit of the TRC has been "woven into the political, economic and social structures that have independently begun to formulate new 'post-apartheid' truths and representations" (Stanley 2001, 543). This became apparent during the Marikana Massacre, when a built-up stand-off between government and mine owners on the one hand and striking miners on the other culminated in a series of conflicts at the Lonmin Mine in Marikana, North West Province. Between 11 and 16 August 2012, a stand-off emerged, striking mine workers facing Lonmin security, police and members of the National Union of Mine Workers. After a period of shooting live ammunition, more than 44 people died, more than 70 were injured, and 250 were arrested (South African Government 2015). On 16 August, an especially brutal pushback occurred from the police, when they started shooting into the crowd with assault rifles, killing 34 miners in the process. It was the most violent oppression of civilians by armed forces since the 1960 Sharpville Massacre half a century before.

Subsequently, the president at the time, Jacob Zuma, called for a commission of inquiry, a type of fact-finding procedure to unveil the truth of the events at Marikana, chaired by Judge Ian Farlam. A report of the findings was produced in 2015, suggesting that the series of increasingly violent, unprotected strikes in neighbouring mines leading up to the massacre was to blame. The report recommended, among other things, that the Director of Public Prosecutions investigate the conduct and culpability of miners during the conflict (this process is, to date, still on-going). It recommended that public policing be reformed to avoid a repeat of this amount of death and injury in future, and found that Lonmin was at least partly to blame (high-ranking government officials and ministers were absolved). Ultimately, labour relations in the mining sector were not reformed, but the focus fell on security and punishment.

These three events – the TRC, Marikana, Life Esidimeni – were very much assaults on the ANC's political and moral legitimacy to rule, undermining the promises made during the "Mandela Decade" (Sitas 2010), and seriously questioned the achievement of social justice for the vulnerable and marginalised. A thread that goes through these three events is the public manner in which it was sought to be resolved. The particular manner of and space where these processes took place is significant, and start to open our understanding about the pursuit of justice for human rights abuses in post-apartheid South Africa. In the next section, the public nature and associated appearances of the Life Esidimeni arbitration process is briefly discussed through a lens of the public sphere.

Justice in a public sphere

Seeking justice in a public space, where all can access the facts presented is a vital (though also limited) aspect of democracy and citizenship: "Circulation of information and access to public venues where one can criticize government officials are vital for liberal democratic governance" (Adut 2012, 257). When relating the public sphere, one is reminded of Habermas, in his conception of the public sphere as a physical or virtual realm of social life where public opinions are formed, open (in principle at least) to all citizens, where conversations about the common good are formed (Habermas 1991). Importantly, for the public sphere to achieve rational consensus, the discourse needs to be universal, without the influences of class, religion, ethnicity and other related classifications. Ari Adut takes inspiration from this position, but argues that – especially in contemporary times – the public sphere is a realm of appearances (not as Habermas argued, one of citizenship), with a central event of spectacle, rather than of dialogue (Adut 2018). In this sense, South Africa's public displays of justice seeking (under the assumption of truth as vehicle for justice) becomes a study in the "semiotics of general visibility". Adut uses the idea of public scandal, "a quintessential public event", to illustrate this – something which Life Esidimeni very much was. He refers to …

an episodic event that is occasioned by the publicization of a real or alleged transgression to a negatively oriented audience."

Insofar as the underlying function of an event in the public sphere provides a space where signs and symbols designate connections between content and the audience. A key consideration here is access – physical (being there in person), representational (being represented in a public space by name, image, sound or words), and sensory access (the availability of content to the public's senses) (Adut 2012). The Life Esidimeni saga involved all three in different respects: The arbitration process provided physical access to a limited number of the public, victim's families and their representation, and various state and non-state actors; this process was also live streamed via internet video sites, television news channels, and the event, as well as the Ombud Report and various statements by stakeholders were relayed on various news and social media platforms; the victims themselves were represented by narratives provided by their families. The public participated in the dissemination of the content of the Life Esidimeni discourse, mediated through news and social media (as opposed to have direct exposure (Adut 2018). The underlying function of the publicness of the arbitration process, the Ombud Report and the subsequent communications between parties was to expose truth, a truth that is perceived as something that can only be unearthed in a public space through confession and judgement. In this vein, the public sphere is a space of appearances: "in public, we are simply what we seem to be". Internal states matter much less than appearances in spectators' judgement (Adut 2012). As in the case of the TRC (and arguably, in the case of the Marikana report), the truth was one of appearances, something that only lifts the veil to a limited extent.

Another dimension to consider here is publicity, which is sometimes used opportunistically to the derogation of others. This is particularly relevant in the political arena, where political actors publicise the scandals of their opponents to generate publicity, sometimes through provocative, moral attacks (Adut 2012). This kind of political opportunism was perhaps best exemplified by the Democratic Alliance's 2019 election campaign, that included the promotion of the slogan "The ANC is killing us". This strategy included erecting a controversial billboard in Johannesburg city centre with the names of people who died during the Marikana massacre, the Life Esidimeni scandal and the numerous children who have drowned in pit toilets in socioeconomically deprived areas (a key challenge to the ANC's legitimacy to rule as a voice for the people). The strategy somewhat backfired when the families of the Life Esidimeni victims and others voiced their disapproval of using the memory of the dead in a political stunt, inferring support from the victims' families. Ultimately, "we cannot make sense of scandal independent of the semiotics of general visibility" (Adut 2012, 256). The consequences suffered by actors embroiled in scandal are very much tethered to how they appear in public, and because they often represent wider groups, the group might also suffer. Qedani Mahlangu's reluctance to appear at the arbitration hearings, and the focus on her subsequent unrepentance and unwillingness to accept blame vilified her in public, and personified the failings of the post-apartheid ANC government. Her reinstatement into the leadership structures of the ANC drove this point home, and underlined the strong party ethos of loyalty to party members as a principle and over-riding value above all else.

The public sphere is superficial, reducing actors to appearances and types; it has an "elemental inauthenticity", and "all moral qualities displayed in public, except maybe courage, are inherently disputable" (Adut 2018, 142). Consider that, in terms of access, no actual, direct voice from people with severe mental and neurological conditions was part of this process, only representation. The judgement of the audience is also affected: the knowledge that others are experiencing the same emotional response as we are, intensifies the experience (Adut 2012). Again, similar to the TRC, the tragic narratives of victim's life stories filled the public with sorrow; gruesome details of the number and nature of deaths filled us with horror; and accounts of unrepentant, incompetent and arrogant state officials filled us with anger. This is not to say that public reactions were without merit, but rather that it only represented a part-truth. In reality, thousands of people with severe mental and neurological conditions suffer similar fates to those in the Life Esidimeni saga, even as this is being written. The public sphere, its appearances and publicity, does not guarantee justice – it can easily warp truth, and disregard certain facts, individuals and groups (Adut 2012).

Ultimately, the centrality of appearances in the public sphere does not only elicit moral judgement, but also aesthetic judgement. State power to judge is only properly catalysed when it is seen by civil society, if it is open for all to see (Adut 2018). Aesthetic appearances have become a central consideration in the ways in which judgement and justice are pursued in post-apartheid South Africa; arbitration processes occur in the public, framing the pursuit and achievement of justice in a decentralised, collective and democratic way. However, this gives a false sense of contentment. In reality, the structures and processes within which the actions of actors are embedded continue, justice remains out of reach, and people with severe mental and neurological conditions continue to suffer in various ways on a daily basis.

Towards a distributive justice

The basic principles of justice transcend all other considerations and pierce all dimensions of the social fabric (Rawls 1999). This being said, far be it from the remit of this book to explore the depth and breadth of justice in the wake of Life Esidimeni. Though, we could perhaps lay the grounds for future investigation. In this vein, there is potential in exploring how justice could better be served in a distributive sense, following Rawls. Accordingly, justice for the people with severe mental and neurological conditions who suffered and died during the Gauteng Mental Marathon Project can be achieved by applying the two principles of justice: (1) Did the victims have an equal right to the most extensive scheme of equal liberties, compared to a scheme of equal liberties for all, and (2) were the social and economic inequalities within which they were immersed subject to fair equality of opportunity, and arranged in such a way that they are to the greatest benefit of the least advantaged (Rawls 1971). It is important to note that, by equality, we mean not only formally and legally, but substantively. The basic position of people, no matter their positions in society, their forms of capital, their status within any social structures, is that all are equal (Rawls 1999). South Africa's Constitution and various legal instruments are widely respected for highlighting the ideal of equal opportunity, including the Mental Health Care Act; as Life Esidimeni and other failures demonstrated though, formal legal equality is not enough.

If we had pursued the Gauteng Mental Marathon Project behind a veil of ignorance (a philosophical tool employed by Rawls to hypothesise whether an action would lead to the maximum benefit of the worst off in society if one is completely oblivious of a person's background, social standing or any other form of status or rank), then it most certainly would not have happened. The absence of community support, the extremely slim chance that the move would benefit the participants, would render any action unjust. Apart from these considerations, we should keep in mind that the arbitration processes in the Life Esidimeni saga largely focused on the families of victims, and not the victims themselves. The families were provided with an opportunity to discuss their pain and suffering, and to participate in the truth-telling process. They ultimately were beneficiaries of substantial financial compensation, and became an important civic group that continued to apply pressure to government. We should not however forget that the primary victims of this saga were the people who suffered and died during and after the transfer, and they represent a group that has suffered the brunt of societal marginalisation for centuries.

In this way, we can go a step further, by claiming that true justice in equality can only be achieved if radical and far-reaching systems reform takes place, to the extent that the relative positions of people with severe mental and neurological conditions maximise their well-being. True justice in Life Esidimeni would mean that, on top of retribution and repatriation, we would go a step further and reform the system in such a way that would prevent future failures. Again, this will not be achieved by policy and legislation alone, but would potentially require strong leadership and substantial political empowerment of people with severe mental and neurological conditions, their families and caretakers, as well as their neighbourhoods and communities. The permeability of the boundaries between state and non-state, between public and private, requires that any kind of differentiation should be firmly embedded in the political will of citizens in order to legitimise any claims they make to "fair value" of their liberties (Habermas 1995). In other words, the locus of power needs to be firmly seated in communities. When there is capacity to generate social goods for some, fairness would call on us to distribute that good to all, especially to the most vulnerable (Ikkos, Boardman,

& Zigmond 2006). The Rawlsian principle of difference is critical, as – especially in the case of people with severe mental and neurological conditions – unjustly hurt their self-respect by not being adequately recognised (Rawls 1999). The difference principle and the primary social good of self-respect are closely tied together, and is of particular relevance. Self-esteem is a primary social good because it affirms the degree to which equal citizenship has been achieved. Social good are, in this sense, things needed by citizens to live as free and equal persons, and include the social bases of self-respect, institutional mechanisms that personal promote self-worth (Rawls 2001). Richard Sennett (2003) contends that inequalities severely disrupt the pillars of respect (to help others, to make something of yourself, to care for yourself), which frames critical dimensions of care in terms of severe mental and neurological conditions. A central ideal in the welfare state is that we should help and respect others, while also promoting autonomy of care. These are not new principles in the mental health sciences, but when they are framed as elements of social justice rather than therapeutic mechanisms, its importance becomes all the more pressing. There is probably no more well-described root cause for modern day inequality than the neoliberal brand of capitalism, pervasive in global development trajectories over the past half century. The economistic values inscribed in neoliberal approaches tend to override considerations of equal liberty of people with severe mental and neurological conditions. These effects have been hinted at in thus far, but a more focused discussion is warranted.

Note

1 Deinstitutionalisation is often framed as a result of a growing academic and cultural critique of psychiatry and institutionalisation during the 1960–1980 period, especially in the United States. Critique by noted psychiatrists such as Thomas Szaz, David Cooper and RD Laing, research by social scientists such as Erving Goffman and David Rosenhan, and post-structural critiques from people like Michel Foucault attacked the credibility of psychiatry as a science, and institutionalisation and a health care strategy. On a more mainstream level, films such as *Shock Corridor*, *One Flew Over the Cuckoo's Nest* and *Titicut Follies* focused on emotive visual depictions of cruelty to institutionalised psychiatric patients, adding a cultural stream of critique to academic debates. The result was a political movement to shut down psychiatric institutions in a wide-scale reform strategy which, in the United States at least, led to many people suffering from severe mental and neurological conditions becoming homeless or imprisoned, on top of increasing morbidity and mortality. For a detailed account of this process, as well as the lessons learnt for mental health care, see David Mechanic's *Inescapable Decisions: The Imperatives of Health Reform* (1994) and *Deinstitutionalisation: An Appraisal of Reform* (1990); David Rochefort's *From Poorhouses to Homelessness: Policy Analysis and Mental Health care* (1997); Howard Goldman and Joseph Morrisey's *The Alchemy of Mental Health Policy: Homelessness and the Fourth Cycle of Reform* (1985), and George Paulson's *Closing the Asylums* (2012).

7 Neoliberal mental health care in post-apartheid South Africa

Introduction

There is a tendency to lay blame for specific atrocities and poor health and socioeconomic outcomes in general at the feet of neoliberalism and its various ills, and not only from the corners of critical scholarship. Indeed, a quick search in EbscoHost, a meta search engine for scholarly work, produces 13,849 hits, from 1960 to the present day – and this only included the terms "neoliberalism or neoliberal or neoliberal policy" in the titles of published studies. A similar search in PubMed – one of the most trusted medical and health databases of scholarly work – suggests that studies with "neoliberalism" or "neoliberal" in its title grew from an average of 4 per year from 1991 to 2007, to 19 per year from 2008 to 2020 (the first half of 2020 already produced 22). This tendency has also proliferated in attempts to make sense of South Africa's post-apartheid dynamics, including health and health care. Nonetheless, apart from a select few examples (e.g. Ornellas & Engelbrecht 2018), a critical look at the relationship between South Africa's broader socioeconomic and political landscape and mental health system reform has not yet been fully explored. As a key partner in the Movement for Global Mental Health, South Africa has been relatively cut out of critique that have been levelled at the Movement on a global scale. Often relying on critical theory as a starting point, especially various forms of critical race and anti-psychiatry approaches, these include arguing that global mental health system strengthening that focus efforts in LMICs are a form of psychiatric imperialism, that such efforts promote the global reach of pharmaceutical industries, or simply a manifestation of global neoliberal forces (Cosgrove & Karter 2018). Such arguments are ongoing, without resolution, and important. In the present case though, despite a fairly large body of literature on the ways in which neoliberalism has shaped South Africa's post-apartheid reality (see, for instance, the works of Ben Fine, Gillian Hart, Nicoli Nattrass, Sampie Terblanche and Patrick Bond – among many others), there is a need to explore this more, especially given the relative sterility with which such questions have been treated in local mental health care scholarship. In this chapter, we start to disentangle the possibly precarious relationship between South Africa's presupposed neoliberal dynamics and the structuring of public mental health care.

What do we mean by neoliberalism?

We need to pause and first consider the vague nature of the term "neoliberalism". Its use in popular media, especially following times of crisis, has been malleable in that it has been used to describe a range of different ills associated with late modernism (often used interchangeably with associated terms such as "capitalism", "elitism" and "free market economics"). Nikolas Rose suggests that an uncritical adoption of terms such as governmentality and neoliberalism to different contexts, purely in its Anglo-Foucauldian forms, undermine the power of such concepts to better understand social phenomena (Carvalho 2015). Here, Gillian Hart proves valuable, by critically examining contradicting forces in the post-apartheid period through a (largely Marxist) lens that adopts Gramsci, Foucault and more inductive, bottom-up considerations of South African politics. Rather than simply designating the South African context as "neoliberal", we should rather attempt to expose the number of examples of neoliberal rationalities that emerge in the political sphere (Gillian Hart 2008). Neoliberalism has become more than a mere type of economic policy that follows the Washington Consensus, but rather a set of tactics and strategies aimed at diffusing market competition throughout the social sphere. Neoliberalism has been understood as a set of political and economic ideas in the spirit of monetarism; as institutions, policies and practices that embody and operationalise this spirit; as a class-based attack against the working class in step with capital motivations; and as a form of social, economic and political reproduction through financialisaton, in an advanced stage of capitalism (Fine & Saad-Filho 2017). By recasting the liberal economic commitment to individualism in terms of market competition (Bowsher 2020), neoliberalism is also a form of governance, where subjects are developed into enterprising units to fit into and reproduce the over-riding schema of market-driven logic, what was referred to by Foucault as Homo Oeconomicus (Foucault 2008). Loïc Wacquant has an especially relevant definition of neoliberalism, that has roughly been followed in this book. Accordingly, neoliberalism is "a transnational political project aiming to remake the nexus of market, state, and citizenship from above", articulating the institutional logics of (1) economic deregulation, (2) welfare state devolution, retraction, and recomposition, (3) an expansive, intrusive, and proactive penal apparatus, and (4) the cultural trope of individual responsibility (Wacquant 2010, 213). However, accounts of South Africa being at the mercy of the global neoliberal forces of the IMF, the World Bank and other related species, is insufficient and inaccurate. GEAR is unquestionably neoliberal in nature, allowing for much tighter state control over non-state entities and promoting self-governing principles through its message of self-entrepreneurship (Gillian Hart 2008). This being said, its deployment and aftermath suggest more nuance, and requires a consideration of politics amidst the powerful discourses of struggle and liberation. Nonetheless, "top-down" assumptions in approaches to neoliberalism require contestation, and accordingly, in an epistemological vein, we are treating neoliberalism as a type of discourse, where neoliberalism can be "always and only understood as representations through the performative repercussions of discourse", meaning that it is neither "top-down" nor "bottom-up", but rather an iterative, circuitous process (Springer 2012, 142).

Neoliberalism therefore does not only mean pro-market policies such as GEAR, or the privatisation of South Africa's health care by various legal instruments, nor only the involvement of the International Monetary Fund and the World Bank in the 1990s, but also to the ways in which certain structures are routinely reproduced by us as citizens. A proper conceptualisation of neoliberalism, especially in its forms in the South African sense, requires linking class-based, economic approaches, with neoliberalism as a form of governmentality and hegemony (Gillian Hart 2008). Critically, neoliberalism tends to differentiate, measure and judge what is of value and what is not, which amplifies inequalities:

> Whenever an order is manufactured and value is extracted, that which is deemed valueless is made redundant. It is forced to lose its face and its name, that which gives substance to the signifier, and to wear a mask. This does not simply apply to objects. It applies to people as well.
>
> (Mbembe 2019, 158)

Following many tendencies exhibited by the crown jewel of neoliberal states, the United States, instances of neoliberal strategizing are plentiful in South Africa, including privatised health care, security, education and transport; prepaid water and electricity meters; the persisted push to introduce biometrics into social grants management; and an increasingly heavy encompassing of CSOs into the state sphere. However, how did neoliberalism – if at all – influence the structure and nature of post-apartheid mental health care? What follows are brief considerations of specific neoliberal dimensions that have emerged throughout discussions in this book thus far, in no particular order, nor rank.

Shifting responsibility to civil society

Here, there are two main points to consider, both of which are central tenets of neoliberal strategizing. First, there is a tendency to shift services and mandates that are generally viewed as the responsibility of the state, to that of business and civil society. The configuration set out in Chapter 2, where public mental health care is primarily provided by the state and funded by tax flows, supported by civil society and for-profit service providers, changes to shift (even if only slightly) the locus of responsibility away from the state. This has often been interpreted in a misleading way, to mean that neoliberalism equals large-scale privatisation. Neoliberalism however, does not mean a complete retraction of the state. The state provides the legal and regulative architecture for market-oriented logic to proliferate (Wacquant 2009a). Wendy Brown (2003) reminds us that (1) through social, economic, education and penal policy, the state responds to market needs; (2) the state is activated by a deep market rationality, that transcends profitability to include cost-benefit as the guiding principle for all practices ("the state must not simply concern itself with the market but think and behave like a market actor across all of its functions, including law"); the state is responsible for and legitimised by its ability to foster and drive economic growth.

For a while now, the responsibility for people with severe mental and neurological conditions has been taken up by hundreds of CSOs, with different capacities, motivations and reach. The degree of partnership and engagement with state bodies differ substantially across different settings in the country, and their regulation and funding are contingent on provincial government offices' budgeting and prioritisation. Importantly, this does not affect the degree to which CSOs fall under state power, and there are numerous examples of conflict between state and CSOs. This was exemplified by the NAWONGO case (discussed in Chapter 4), but many other examples arise. Recently, this was demonstrated vividly by struggles between the state and CSOs for the distribution of food and basic support to impoverished populations during the COVID-19 crisis. During level four of South Africa's lockdown response to the global COVID-19 pandemic, reports emerged that several communities were suffering from poverty and hunger related to an almost complete cease of the formal economy. This was underlined by indications that some hospitals started seeing a rise in malnutrition cases among children, a political point of conflict between the country's scientific community and the state. There was a surge in community grass roots mobilisation to address food insecurity, ranging from small self-funded soup kitchens to larger initiatives that had lines as long as 3km to receive food parcels. The closure of schools meant that the largest food distribution programme in Africa – the National School Nutrition Programme that provides daily meals to nine million children – was suspended. Effectively, this meant that "just as the need for food escalated, the state locked the doors of its food cupboard and walked away" (Seekings 2020). Within this context, the DoSD attempted to centralise and regulate the flow of food to communities in need, which was met with serious backlash from CSOs. In response, DoSD minister Lindiwe Zulu reverted to the Non-profit Organisations Act, stating that the DoSD is mandated by this act to ensure food security for the vulnerable, but added that reports of overcrowding at distribution points broke infection control regulations, and argued that the uncoordinated nature of the distribution process promoted infection. She called on CSOs "to work jointly with the government to ensure that there is a coordinated response and to eliminate opportunities for corruption and manipulation of these efforts" (News24 2020). Some organisations such as 1000Women1Voice reached out to the international community through the United Nations Women, for help to stop such regulations from being put in place. Others turned to the courts, and the Western Cape High Court instructed the DoSD and national police service that they could not hamper food distribution efforts by CSOs. This flashpoint was not rooted in fears of poor infection control at food distribution sites, but rather speaks to a threat of ANC legitimacy in its most important voter base, namely poor, marginalised communities that are severely dependent on the grants system. This narrative was summarised well by Jeremy Seekings, who remarked that the state has exhibited "commandist instincts", highlighting a discourse of domination and control:

> The name of the "National (Coronavirus) Command Council", Minister of Police Cele's militaristic instructions to the police to criminalise minor infringements of lockdown regulations, Minister of Trade and Industry Patel's micro-regulation of business and 'Disaster' Minister Dlamini-Zuma's obsession with smoking are mirrored in the Minister of Social Development's attempts to control the distribution of food.
>
> (Seekings 2020)

Indeed, the fight for control over different forms of public goods in the bureaucratic field has been telling. Welfare services are paramount public goods, since it provides a moral capacity required in sustaining the legitimacy to lead and control. Moving the responsibility for people living with severe mental and neurological conditions from the for-profit private sphere to civil society speaks to ANC policy to contain, to keep in-house services to specific populations. Similar to early attempts of the DoSD to manage the SASSA distribution system in-house via biometrics, a contract that ultimately fell to the Post Office, the DoH attempted to move the responsibility and care for people with severe mental and neurological conditions "in-house" to CSOs. Here, it is meant that CSOs providing mental health care have become so dependent on government funding, that they have lost much of the very thing that makes them so valuable, namely their proximity to community needs. The regulation system put in place, both by the DoH and DoSD, are constraining to say the least, and the latest DoH draft regulations for CSOs caring for people with severe mental and neurological conditions reflect an almost overbearing degree of health and safety protocols that has to be met – including building codes, safety markings etc. – much like hospital inspections. These biomedically-led regulations set an extraordinarily high bar for CSOs to reach in order to receive state funding. It further entrenches a system that insists on measurement and indicators – reigning in and depoliticising CSOs' strategizing capabilities (Mitlin et al. 2007). Market-led relations and increasing commercialisation may threaten the core values of civil society: corporate human resourcing rather than volunteerism; financial accountability rather than community accountability; and dependence rather that autonomy. Though Wacquant's (2009a) phrasing might seem harsh, his understanding of CSOs as "creatures of the state" under neoliberal times is on point.

Costs and value

The claim that the Life Esidimeni beneficiaries' care was excessive was thoroughly debunked, but it ties in well with a critical point of conflict between the state and CSOs: what is caring for a person with severe mental and neurological conditions worth? This needs to be considered against the background of South Africa's particular welfare state, which is not entirely neoliberal, especially in the American sense. The neoliberal effects of welfare retrenchment and, in parallel, punitive laws and policies – very much the penal state of the United States – on health outcomes are well-known (Nosrati & Marmot 2019). It could be argued that, in a neoliberal context where welfare support is reduced by the state, forcing CSOs to respond to local communities by filling the gap left by agencies such as SASSA. This certainly seems to be the case in terms of community mental health care in many parts of South Africa. However, the neoliberal tendency of contracted welfarism does not completely hold water here, given that social spending has been high relative to other countries. South Africa spent R69,454 million on cash payments for social protection in 2007/2008, which increased to R164,947 million in 2018/2019. Of these amounts, R15,379 million was spent on sickness and disability in 2008/2009, and R20,923 million in 2018/2019. Proportionally, these amounts remained relatively stable: In 2018/2019, social protection constituted 11.3% of total cash transfers, down from 12.2% in 2008/2009 (Statistics South Africa 2009, 2019). Instead of following the key pillars of economic growth, namely capital accumulation, expanding labour demand, and technology growth, the post-apartheid strategy has been to prioritise redistribution ahead of faster economic growth (Fedderke 2009). From 1994 to 2008 there was a dramatic increase in government expenditure on social security and welfare, an increase from 1% to 4% of GDP – among the most generous in LMIC categories. Importantly, this was not a mere circumstance of ANC generosity, but was made possible by a decline in requirements of debt servicing that resulted in a smaller proportion of GDP spent on government debt interest payments. Welfare expansion was therefore made possible by monetary and fiscal policy (Fedderke 2009). Nonetheless, freeing up the budget for welfare expansion was no fluke, and had to occur to the detriment of other programmes (such as defence). Why was there such an extraordinary expansion? Patrick Bond's "talk left walk right" metaphor to expose internal contradictions in ANC policy (Bond 2014) is of value here, as is Gillian Hart's work on the ANC's contradicting processes of de-nationalisation and re-nationalisation in attempts to sustain hegemonic power (Gillian Hart 2014). She highlights that ANC further had – and to some extent still do – a substantial problem of contradicting ideologies, motivations and approaches. This is illuminated by protracted tensions between two approaches: (1) Responsibility, fiscal discipline and efficiency, and (2) local participation, democracy and social justice (Gillian Hart 2008). The outcomes of the TRC, Marikana and Life Esidimeni cases all allude to this tension in one way or another.

Hart explores South Africa's post-apartheid landscape by highlighting key events that expose deeper movements in the political sphere. A key event was the Bredell land occupation in 2001, where thousands of impoverished people from the township of Tembisa bought plots of land at US$3 each from the Pan Africanist Congress of Azania and proceeded to move into the area, on South Africa's East Rand mining belt, owned by the state and various private companies. The occupants were forcefully evicted, and Hart notes the ironic declaration from the Minister of Land and Agricultural Affairs that "these people must go back where they came from" (ironic, because the ANC replaced an apartheid government that actively promoted forceful evictions, under the guise of liberation). Much like Marikana after that, and now, Life Esidimeni, the Bredell exposed a deep moral crisis in the post-apartheid state. It spurred on significant bottom-up counter movements, set against neoliberal capitalism, the ripples of which were felt in instances beyond South Africa. In the years following this event, Mbeki's government clamped down on what was perceived to be neoliberal forces, and capitalist threats from high-income, foreign regions. They also substantially increased welfare spending on the Child Support Grant and poverty reduction in municipalities. Here, Hart notes a governmentality strategy, namely that, by adopting specific, strategically aimed social assistance policies instead of a more universal basic income grant, leverage was gained over the behaviour of key populations (Gillian Hart 2008). The kind of leverage has emerged again in the wake of the COVID-19 outbreak, where the state announced a Special COVID-19 Social Relief of Distress grant, an amount of R350 per month until October 2020, payable to all without any job, income of other forms of social assistance.

The power of liberation discourse receives moral impetus by way of real connections with embodied experiences, subjective histories and meanings of racist oppression and, importantly, struggle against such domination. The ANC succeeds in perpetuating their hegemonic project by driving nationalist discourses and here their true power lies, namely their ability to articulate these discourses among the populace. This is also a vulnerability, because the success of such a narrative depends heavily on an ability to deliver, and this in part explains the extreme frequency of service delivery protests (to the degree that it becomes banal, and almost loses its edge). However, by invoking the emotional pull of concepts such as freedom, justice and liberation, the use of nationalism can easily be turned around to highlight betrayal (Gillian Hart 2008). The eviction of occupants at Bredell, the killing of miners at Marikana, the deaths of Life Esidimeni patients are not once-off incidents nor crimes committed by isolated state agents, but acts of betrayal in the pact made with the people (Gillian Hart 2015). This betrayal no doubt echoes the "original treason", the failure to achieve social justice through the TRC.

The local–global nexus of capital

In describing the Marikana incident, Piketty (2014) is deliberate in stating that the mine in question belonged to the London-based stockholders of

Lonmin, Inc. Hart (2012, 2014) draws our attention to the importance of capital flight in post-apartheid South Africa, detailing how tensions between adopting the lures of global neoliberalism and holding on to power through the use of nationalism has characterised the ANC trajectory. In the same vein, there are potentially important links between global capital and local mental health care arenas. In the NAWONGO case, the outcomes of the court decision were instrumentally decided by KPMG, one of the so-called "Big Four" global auditing firms with a presence in 147 countries. Life Health care, the company with which the Life Esidimeni deal was signed, has moved much of its focus to foreign markets and invests heavily in diagnostic technologies abroad (they currently own UK-based diagnostic company Alliance Medical). In the SASSA case, the fallout with Cash Paymaster Services signalled a desire to draw from Net1's Universal Electronic Payment System (UEPS), a system using biometric monitoring through an electronic card in partnership with banks and governments towards managing social grant payments. This very obviously echoes what Nikolas Rose and Peter Miller meant by governmentality during advanced liberalism. Here, they describe governance over subjects becoming replaced by governmentality, a form of self-governance that allows a mapping of multiple centres of calculation and authority that traverse and link up personal, social and economic life (Miller & Rose 2008), with an aim to create people who are "capable of bearing a kind of regulated freedom" (Rose & Miller 2010b, 174). While it cannot be claimed that advanced liberal governmentality has infused into South Africa's mental health care system to the extent that it can be empirically and routinely described, there certainly have been indications of such a possibility. An important consideration here is the centrality of counting, of differentiation, that has become a feature of social welfare. We should consider now that, as suggested in the NAWONGO case, that people with severe mental and neurological conditions are prioritised or deprioritised within this distribution system, in a differential frame guided by the accounting sciences. This brings us to the next issue, namely the value of a human being with severe mental and neurological conditions in contemporary times.

The value of people with severe mental and neurological conditions

Importantly, and this is a point that was underlined in both the NAWONGO and Life Esidimeni cases, these systems give value to categories of people in line with a neoliberal climate. Under these settings, people with severe mental and neurological conditions have been framed as "financially burdensome", as "costly bodies" consuming scarce resources without providing anything in return, an internalised responsibilisation that problematise dependency through an association with lost productivity (Rotarou & Sakellariou 2017). Mbembe notes that neoliberalism blurs the edges between human subjects and physical objects, that it makes it possible to determine and separate "what is useful from waste, from the detrituses" (p. 158), that gives an economic value to physical bodies, so that it can be measured, quantified, and priced

(Mbembe, 2019). He further muses that democracies perhaps always allow for the possibility of "a set of people who, in one way or another, are regarded as pertaining to the foreigner, members of a surplus population, undesirables of whom one hopes to be rid, and who, in this way, must be left 'completely or partially without rights'" (p. 42). He suggests that, in such spaces, "sovereignty means the capacity to define who matters and who does not, who is *disposable* and who is not" (Mbembe 2019, 80).

Mbembe's thinking here is an amalgamation of Fanon and, particularly relevant here, Foucault. Foucault's work on biopolitics in tandem with a critique of American neoliberalism was particularly well unpacked in a public lecture series at Birkbeck College, University of London, in 2011. The conference theme was "Reflecting on 20 years of The Foucault Effect: Studies in Governmentality", a reflection on the very influential book that very much expanded the Anglicisation of governmentality and biopolitics (https://backdoorbroadcasting.net/tag/the-birkbeck-centre-for-law-and-the-humanities/). Two lectures were particularly relevant for our argument here: Jonathan Simon's *From the Medical Model to the Humanitarian Crisis Model: California's Prison Health Crisis and the Future of Imprisonment* (Simon 2011), and Bernard Harcourt's *The Punitive Order: Free Markets, Neoliberalism, and Mass Incarceration in the United States* (Harcourt 2011). They built on a narrative that suggested that the United States' free market conditions, and privatisation of the prison system, led to conditions where the bodies of (mostly black, poor) socioeconomically marginalised people are incentivised, governed and managed by this neoliberal justice system. The original purpose of punishment falls away to become a form of economic activity, where specific population groups become a form of capital unto themselves. Marx's (1977, 509) notion that "Man can only live if he produces means of subsistence, but he can only produce these means if he holds the means of production, the material conditions of labour" begs the question, what then of those who are physically, mentally or otherwise unable to hold a means of production in a market-driven world? Their lack of inherent value is aggravated by wide-scale disinvestment in the education, housing and health of mostly urban, inner city minorities, which provides a steady supply of bodies for the prison system to turn a profit and expand by cramming more prisoners into existing spaces and building new prisons to cater for the neoliberal norm of market over subjective individual value. Elsewhere, Harcourt (2015) unpacks this idea further, situating the United States' mass incarceration within a longer trajectory of excessive punishment meted out by the state – slavery, Jim Crow laws, mass internment of Japanese-Americans during World War II, and mass institutionalisation of mental patients in asylums up until the 1950s. Reaganism strongly promoted faith in market deregulation and, along with it, theories of human capital that resulted in radical disinvestment in certain populations (mostly racial and ethnic minorities) and reinvestment in others (middle-class prison labour). Ultimately,

> new notions of human capital are important here, and are different: they facilitate a politics at home that treats people as human capital *some of whom are worth the investment, and others not*. It gives way to governmental policies that differentiate between good and bad human investments. And politics soon becomes the art of discerning in whom to invest.
>
> (Harcourt 2015)

Loïc Wacquant explored such strategies of the "neoliberal Leviathan" in his studies of the governance of the urban poor in the US, where populations are stratified and codified, a process during which poor, black urban populations often come second (Wacquant 2009a, 2009b). Importantly, while many neo-liberal tropes suggest less state intervention in favour of unregulated and free markets, Wacquant showed how a variety of state apparatuses are used to manage vulnerable population by applying a market-oriented logic and legal tools to that management (Wacquant 2009a).

The state fosters legitimacy by claiming to provide for the well-being of the population, driven by an instrumental economic rationality of costs and benefits (Chatterjee 2004). Under these conditions, people living with severe mental and neurological conditions – who have little chance of entering and remaining in the labour market – personifies Homo Sacer, the cast out, where "bare life" becomes the authentic subject of politics (Agamben 1998). They become subjects of Homo Economicus, essentially existing under a "spectre of uselessness", a challenge to the state provision of welfare benefits (Sennet 2014). The state provides the infrastructure that fosters supportive conditions for the working of quasi-markets (Carvalho 2015), and the framing of this group, in an incredibly cold and aloof way, as "useless", transforms them into forms of capital, objects of economic rationalities. Their commodification is often not even very subtle. Officially aiming to improve their quality of life through welfare support, the SASSA disability grant system transforms its recipients into modalities for income which, in socioeconomically marginalised and desperate families, depersonifies the beneficiary and turns him/her into a source of income. Here, we need to make it clear that welfare support is in itself not malevolent but, in the absence of parallel investments into social systems, the chances of exploitation are much higher. We see this most arrestingly in the NAWONGO case where the application of auditing technologies resulted in a ranking of welfare recipients purely in terms of cost-benefit terms. The inherent capital of people with severe mental and neurological conditions were ranked and compared against other "programmes", such as geriatric care and care for vulnerable and orphaned children. The decision about where to invest is guided by the costs of need (the "need" here is also debatable, and requires interrogation), with an inherent expectation of returns. In the Life Esidimeni Ombud Report, there was an analysis conducted that delineates costs associated for the care per person per day in private versus public hospital, as part of debunking the GDoH's claim that their decision to cease the contract was informed by economics. This decision was telling in that it was claimed that the costs paid for a relatively small group of beneficiaries were too high, that the funds would rather be allocated elsewhere, and the Life Esidimeni patients will be moved to "cheaper" community-based care. Crucially, it would seem that the CSOs were pitted against each other in competition for bodies, as each individual brings with it an amount of income – the victims thus represented little more than cash value. The following excerpt from the Ombud Report refers (Makgoba 2017, 2):

> *frail, disabled and incapacitated patients were transported in inappropriate and inhumane modes of transport, some 'without wheel chairs but tied with bed sheets' to support them; some NGOs rocked up at LE in open 'bakkies' [trucks] to fetch MHCUs [mental health care users] while others chose MCHUs like an 'auction cattle market' despite pre-selection by the GDMH [Gauteng Department of Mental Health] staff; some MCHUs were shuttled around several NGOs; during transfer and after deaths several relatives of patients were still not notified or communicated to timeously; some are still looking for relatives; these conducts were most negligent and reckless and showed a total lack of respect for human dignity, care and human life.*

This unfolded in a mental health system where, as described in Chapter 2, the state subsidises CSOs based on number cared for, and not based on any outcomes related to well-being. Instead, the approach is punitive – CSOs are subjected to regulation with the sword of de-certification hanging over them. Of course, in Life Esidimeni none of the CSOs were certified, and the state could therefore, to some degree at least, move responsibility onto the CSOs without regulating them. On their part, CSOs, weakened in terms of activism, reliant on the state for legitimacy and financial viability, participate in this system and often bend their focus to fit with the state's needs. Ultimately, much like in the US penal system, in South Africa there has been large disinvestment in the community-based care and support for the vulnerable, along with investment in institutionalised care as part of the state's fiscal focus.

A challenge emerges when one compares today's mental health system dynamics with those of the 1960s, where neoliberalism would not normally be applicable (though this is far from definite). Discussions of neoliberalism should therefore be appended by considerations of the historical reverberations of colonialism and imperialism (Gillian Hart 2008). In particular, this means that we need to consider that the stark similarities between the Life Esidimeni case and the 1960 Smith Mitchell and Co fall-out are far from coincidental. The themes have remained depressingly similar: people designated as divergent and requiring intervention are "sold" to non-state entities, who receive cash flow per body per month, live in facilities with woefully, criminally low standards of care, and, in some cases, are drawn into the labour market through protective workshops, under the guise of "keeping busy" or the biomedical parameters of occupational therapy. Importantly, intervention only occurs after substantial death and suffering, exposed by the media, leading to justice in an almost one dimensionally economic sense, but a continuation of the status quo in terms of systems make-up. The racial angle might have ceased in terms of legal and policy status, but in reality, facilities – both state and non-state – caring for people with severe mental and neurological conditions remain, much like in almost every other social programme, racially divided. There are vast differences in terms of resources, both financial and professional, between CSOs that operate through Christian Afrikaner, or British Anglican or Catholic backing, and the CSOs that operate in and provide services to informal settlements and township areas. This is not to say that the two camps focus on particular races in terms of policy, but rather speaks to the persistence of apartheid geographies and the incredibly strong sociocultural divisions that remain in South Africa's health and social systems. A stark reminder of these divisions lies in the aesthetics of mental health facilities. Private hospitals and clinics that provide mental health care for profit are adorned with framed art pieces, soft lighting, and an almost over-supply of mental health professionals of the highest calibre – the settings are almost opulent in comparison to state facilities and CSOs relying on donations and grants. This is a rather obvious statement, and South Africa's inequities are almost over-described (to the degree that such statements lose their power). Nonetheless, the unambiguous differences between private and public mental health care's capital – not just economic capital, but cultural capital – is yet another example of the unrighteousness developing off the confluence of apartheid, colonialism and neoliberal politics.

This brings us to the matter of investment. In his influential work *Capital in the Twenty-First Century*, Thomas Piketty highlighted the notorious Marikana incident of August 2012 (where 34 striking miners were killed by state police forces) as an example of the immense inequalities in the capital-labour split in the modern era, which often result in violent clashes between workers and their economic masters (Piketty 2014). Indecently, in her book "Rethinking the South African Crisis Nationalism, Populism, Hegemony", Gillian Hart (2013) also started with a description of Marikana; though both used the event as a starting point of a critique of capitalism, they proceed from different angles. Here, Marikana serves as an example of investment into human forms of capital in South Africa. Mining companies such as Lonmin invest heavily in private hospitals for their workforce – principally to keep their workforce healthy. This is particularly salient for the management of tuberculosis, a disease rife among the South African mineworker population, and the subject of astounding academic interest and experimentation (Churchyard et al. 2014) AngloGold Ashanti – who operates the Lonmin mine – is in many ways the epitome of the success of global capitalism, operating in eleven countries and listed on five major stock exchanges. Keeping the workforce healthy is a key concern in the reproduction of capital, and in this way investing in the physical bodies of mine workers is tied to profit. Mental health certainly is not a consideration here; people whose ability to work and take part in the economic system is hampered by an illness which often does not have a good prognosis are not worth investing into within the contexts of a global neoliberal marketplace. However, this does not mean that people with debilitating mental conditions are inherently worthless in this system – they become the forms of capital themselves. Let's look again at the United States, where a double act of (1) disinvestment in poor, urban, black minorities, and (2) a parallel investment in a penal system that generates profit out of the numbers of inmates produced by the disinvestment, vividly illustrates the mechanics of a system that places value on, and generates profit from, the objectification of certain populations (Harcourt 2011, 2015; Simon 2011; Wacquant 2008, 2009a, 2009b, 2010). The commodification of people with severe mental and neurological conditions are thus neither unique to South Africa, nor confined to contemporary times. Similar instances where vulnerable populations have been exploited for financial gain can certainly also be found in mental health, and not only in South Africa's Smith Mitchell and Co and Life Esidimeni cases. An infamous example stems from the Duplessis Orphans in Canada during the 1940s and 1950s, where around 20,000 orphans were classified to be "mentally deficient" by the Quebec government and Catholic Church, where economics, politics and psychiatry combined to exploit the bodily integrity of the vulnerable. The Quebec government received large federal subsidies to build hospitals to meet a perceived demand for care, and in return paid the Church much higher subsidies than they would have if the children were merely classified as orphans (psychiatric care meant higher subsidies). Psychiatric state custodians brought in more than twice as much as orphaned ones per head per day. Subsequently, as per the financial incentive, thousands of orphaned children were wrongly classified and committed to atrocious circumstances in 16 psychiatric hospitals run by the Church. However, as in the Smith Mitchell and Co case, the commodified bodies were put to work as well, thereby generating additional income streams (Boucher, Pare, Perry, Sigal, & Ouimet 2008). Exploited subjects like these fundamentally constitute

> reserves of value in the eyes of their owners. ... In the same way as money or again commodities, they served as a medium for all sorts of economic and social transactions. As movable objects and extended matter, theirs was the status of that which circulates, is invested in, and is expended.
>
> (Mbembe 2019, 31)

This entails a flow of capital from taxpayers to private companies, endorsed and supported by the state apparatus who are the legitimate stewards of population health and well-being. We see a similar unfolding in the South African milieu and in the cases described: In the Life Esidimeni case, the GDoH aimed to cut costs spent on the care of people with severe mental and neurological conditions, claiming that the amount spent on the Life Esidimeni contract was unaffordable: "*It is important to note that the Department cannot afford this, the budget allocation which was previously utilised on the said facility will be reprioritised accordingly*" (Mahlangu 2015b). However, as pointed out in the Ombuds Report (Makgoba 2017), this line of reasoning was flawed: Only direct costs related to Life Esidimeni care were calculated, and no feasibility studies or costing exercises were performed towards alternative care options. The costs of R320 per patient per day at Life Esidimeni were below market-related health care costs; average health care costs per patient per day at state-funded Weskoppies, Sterkfontein Cullinan Care and Rehabilitation Centre hospitals were calculated at R1,960.41, R1,386.13 and R1,486.04, respectively. Furthermore, the less obvious costs of health care such as the retransfer and re-admission of patients were not included in the decision. The estimated amount of R112 per patient per day for CSO-based care suggests a rationality grounded in cost-cutting at the detriment of basic human rights (Makgoba 2017, 28):

> *The only means to cut costs in order to adjust to the high hospitalisation expenditure were to provide extremely cheap care to the majority of MHCUs [Mental Health Care Users]. To expect that residential home CTR [Care, Treatment and Rehabilitation] can be provided at just over R 112 per day indicates a lack of understanding of current costs of living and/or a disregard of the human right to dignity and quality care of these MHCUs.*

Ultimately, the neoliberal "competence machine" that generates market-relevant human capital through investments in health, education etc. is inherently differential in its targets (Raffnsøe, Gudmand-Høyer, & Thaning 2016). People with severe mental and neurological conditions are very much excluded from this investment strategy.

The centrality of death

The plight of people with severe mental and neurological conditions are exacerbated when one considers their position in population mortality risk estimates. A growing epidemiological literature that suggests that they constitute a population that are at a substantially higher risk to suffer premature mortality, due to various lifestyle and cardiovascular conditions link to their illness (Charlson et al. 2016; de Mooij et al. 2019; John et al. 2018). A US study estimated that, at a minimum, one in four people with severe mental illness who have an encounter with the police suffer a fatality (Fuller, Lamb, Biasotti, & Snook 2015). The premature death of this population is largely due to social and behavioural drivers – not clinical. While Life Esidimeni illustrated this vulnerability in dramatic fashion, it is by no means a stretch to think of the spaces that are occupied by people with severe mental and neurological conditions as spaces of precarity. Beyond the biopolitics of Foucault and Nikolas Rose, we are confronted by an instance of Achille Mbembe's necropolitics. The state, as custodians of people with mental and neurological conditions, have an ultimate degree of sovereignty over their fates; "To be sovereign is to exert one's control over mortality and to define life as the deployment and manifestation of power" (Mbembe 2019, 66). By holding legal, social and economic power over the contexts of care, the state creates – even if unintentionally – "death worlds", "new and unique forms of social existence in which vast populations are subjected to living conditions that confer upon them the status of the *living dead*" (Mbembe 2019, 132).

Death indeed becomes an important political consideration, as a particular discursive power. There is a particular pressing urgency that accompany the reporting of scandals and tragedies in terms of the amounts, and nature, of death. Mortality rates are a powerful leverage mechanism in global health and humanitarianism. Casualty counts are a key argument for prioritisation, and crisis and progress are both measured in terms of a quantification of life and death. Mortality and morbidity indicators are very much the "currency of international action" (Auchter 2019). Consider the reporting of events like the 2014 Ebola outbreak in West Africa, and more recently, the COVID-19 pandemic, the death toll of which has become a key mechanism for action. The software developed by Johns Hopkins University mapping out the latest figures of the spread and mortality of the virus with large red dots is a particularly vivid reminder of the power of mortality statistics. In mental health, there are often papers in global mental health that cite in their background suicide rates to create a sense of priority and urgency in studying conditions like depression. Suicide is an incredibly important challenge, but surely not the outcome that we should be focusing on when studying mental illness? Death becomes a way to convince the public that an issue is important, but in the process, it papers over issues like prevention in a more structural sense. In this vein, death becomes an important discursive marker. The by-line of the title of the Life Esidimeni Ombud Report was "No Guns: 94+ Silent Deaths and Still Counting", and the whole saga was covered by virtue of how many died, numbers jumping from the 30s to the 90s to 144. It was also not only the numbers of death, but their nature – the discussion of the ways in which the victims died became a point of morbid fascination, and the media ran with flashy headlines and articles detailing the contents of the report and the arbitration process thereafter, focusing on the particularly gruesome instances. The part of the report that dealt with autopsy results became a powerful tool to sell the horror of the event – recall details of death due to dehydration, hunger etc. Ultimately, the focus on death as avoidable outcome overrides any other concerns – the structural elements of poor care, the continuing inhuman conditions within which many people with severe mental and neurological conditions barely survive. Very rarely mention was made during the Life Esidimeni saga of those who did not die, and those who are exploited in other organisations, facilities, and provinces – the focus stayed firmly tuned on the deaths as primary concern.

We are well aware that the media is skewed as interpreting mechanism between events and the public. Daniel Khaneman (2011) explores this notion and suggests that mortality cause estimates are very much distorted by media coverage, as the actual coverage of things that lead to death are intimately intertwined with novelty and poignancy. Media reports of mortality are very much shaped by the nature of what is being reported. Susan Sontag's well-known works on the deeper associations that are drawn by different forms of illness underlines this point: cancer has been associated with repression, depressive states, sensuality, and people who lack passion; tuberculosis has been associated with creativity, and death due to the disease as due to a lack of passion (Sontag 1978); while HIV/AIDS has been associated with judgement of behaviour, a consequence of deviant sexual behaviour (which often translates into homophobic judgement) and decadence (Sontag 1989). Perceptions of and attitudes toward severe mental and neurological conditions have been the subject of thousands of articles, books, art and music, and the body of knowledge on this subject requires a library of its own. The history of ties with godly judgement, and supernatural abilities are well-known, and the persistent lack of success in robustly attempting to pin down root causes for the range of conditions under discussion certainly may have contributed to the tenacity of certain stereotypes. The deinstitutionalisation movement has opened up a lot of mystery associated with severe mental illness, and the advent of community-based mental health care has also brought conceptions of mental illness out from behind the walls of the asylum and into the public sphere, confronting the public with visual proximity to an issue that has traditionally been shamed and hidden (Borinstein 1992). A key assumption in discourses of severe mental and neurological conditions is that their illness is a disability, an impairment that renders them without agency. The individualisation of this assumption is telling, as these subjects become objects requiring intervention and "care". Their subjectivities and resistance are denied existence, and they become perpetual victims. Their death becomes a consequence of their illness, not as a consequence of the broader systems within which they exist. This renders their precarity decidedly moral, tied up in three rationalities (Fassin 2015, xi):

> the welfare state, which protects the subjects from the hazards of life; the penal state, which decides which crime to punish and how, and the liberal state, which mobilizes simultaneously individual rights and individual obligations. In the past decades, the decline of the welfare state has been paralleled by the expansion of the penal state, while the liberal state has appeared as a way to legitimize the former evolution by invoking the responsibility of the subject and to mitigate the latter trend by introducing minimal legal guarantees. This ambiguous moral configuration is a unique feature of the contemporary state.

8 Concluding thoughts

> These and all the other uncountable tuberculous pasts remain our potential futures.
>
> –Helen Bynum, Spitting Blood (2012, 268)

The study of mental health care is tightly wrapped in "the inseparability of the moral, the medical, and the political" (Kleinman 1998, 395). The stakes in reforming mental health care is not only tied to improved clinical, economic and other associated outcomes, but also to the moral imperatives of care. It is no exaggeration to state that people with severe mental and neurological conditions are a marginalised group, perpetually open to what many term "structural violence", with little to no voice and power and agency to change their precarious position on the peripheries of society. Prior to the transfer, 532 patients have lived in Life Esidimeni facilities for 10 years or more, 773 had no contact with their families, 474 had no identification documents, and 217 were categorised "without ID, without family" (Comrie 2016). This is but a microcosm of a population that continues to live in these circumstances as we speak, in South Africa and beyond. In attempting to demystify how the Life Esidimeni tragedy was made possible, Dr Aaron Motsoaledi, testified on 31 January 2018 the following:

> I have been asking myself that question ever since this thing has started, because there is a lot of criminality in this whole thing. And in any criminal activity there is usually a motive. I looked left, right and centre what the motive could have been. … I am afraid it beats me, up to today. And in parliament they even asked me, could the motive have been money. And I said, to subject so many people to what has [they have] been subject [subjected] to until they die, it needs to be billions that we are chasing. I still … so I am puzzled, I honestly don't know, and that is why it is difficult for me.

The Life Esidimeni events lifted the veil of the ways in which modern society "manages", "treats" and "governs" the lives of the vulnerable and the voiceless. Here, there is a body of incredibly valuable and relevant literature that can help us to make more sense of the reasons why the outcomes of people with severe mental illness are often so dire. Neoliberal rationalities have fused with ANC politics and has eroded our collective sense of justice, leading to an evisceration of democratic morality (Brown 2003). South Africa's post-apartheid health system has seen incredible changes, and massive gains have been made in the past three decades. Nonetheless, when engaging with mental illness and its care, one is forced to wonder if we are moving in circles. Whether we have not, despite substantial investment, lobbying and policy change during the past half century, found ourselves back in a version of the workhouses of Victorian times. Foucault's Great Confinement is certainly over (in its physical form, in any case), but perhaps he was accurate in describing deinstitutionalisation as a new form of governance. To be clear – in South Africa at least – deinstitutionalisation and community-based care is still a form of institutionalisation. There simply is no present scenario where people with severe mental and neurological conditions are not institutionalised by the state in some form, and this could be framed as a measure to minimise risk to the community; as a way in which to provide care as part of a human rights imperative; as a part of the welfare industry; or in various other ways. Nonetheless, institutionalisation is firmly inscribed in our society in terms of law, policy and general norm consensus. A more accurate term would be de-hospitalisation, a move away from the asylum model of the early 20th century, towards CSOs that somehow fall in the middle of the spectrum between asylums on the one point and home-based, family-driven care on the other. The goal is to fulfil the range of complex needs of this population (a population which, as pointed out in the first chapter, is far from homogenous though is often treated in this way), in an environment which is unrestrictive and meant to promote well-being and rehabilitation, close to the community where the person is from in order to be close to their family and to destigmatise mental illness and disability. This is to be achieved to the highest degree possible with available funds and resources. Fulfilling the clinical and emotional therapeutic needs on top of making sure that the basic needs of food, shelter and hygiene are achieved, is for many CSOs a daily battle. As for the ideal of less restriction on movement, many CSOs tend to keep close control over their clients – in some cases this involves a rule to not leave the property unaccompanied without prior permission, while in other (especially in less well-resourced CSOs), this involves putting up barbed wire fencing around the property to create a physical barrier between clients and community access (Janse van Rensburg 2018). The problems described here are neither new, nor unique. The challenges in providing adequate and appropriate care and support to people with severe mental and neurological conditions have confounded health systems globally, for centuries. Solutions will not be solely found in care packages or plans, political commitment, increased funding, but requires a shift in values and the ways in which we approach mental health care. Far be it here from providing any recommendations for the improvement of such a complex task, but it might be useful to reflect on areas that could be improved in step with what we have discussed thus far.

First and foremost, we need to consider that the subjective voices of the very people that stand to gain or lose the most in this system, namely those living with severe mental and neurological conditions, are worryingly silent whenever their care is discussed. Their needs and wants were no doubt included, albeit secondarily, in the development of the MHPF and other national frameworks. However, their absence in critically important events between the state and civil society is disquieting. During the NAWONGO case, it is not clear to what degree – if any at all – any of the intended beneficiaries of social support and welfare provided testimony or evidence, or an opinion on the content and nature of service packages designed for them. In the Life Esidimeni post-mortem, it was disturbing how little attention was given to those who survived the ordeal, and the restitution-driven goals of avenging death completely blinded a focus on achieving justice for the living as well. The quarterly intersectoral forums held between state and non-state partners to discuss mental health service provisioning don't include user representation, as in most other governance processes. This remains a massive oversight in our system of care and needs a much stronger insistence on person-centredness. This narrative has been a core part of disability studies scholarship but has remained neglected in discourses around mental health system strengthening.

The imperative to be more person-centred in our approaches to care reform raises an epistemological consideration, namely an argument for "an ethnographic moment" in mental health care, one that focuses on the subjective meanings of suffering and care. This requires us to transcend the economistic language of policy towards prying open spaces for the inclusion of ethnography in how we formulate care (Kleinman 1998). Interactions between service users and service providers is a complex negotiation that frames the ways in which people with severe mental and neurological conditions are perceived, and ultimately, the nature of their care. For instance, discourses of client centredness are differently interpreted by different actors in homelessness support interactions, and client centredness can be associated with discourses of "neediness", "worthiness" and "value", which in turn affects agency and produces different types of homeless client (someone could be branded as resolute, as compliant, or as passive) (Mik-Meyer & Silverman 2019). Similarly, there needs to be much more work done in fully exploring the range of discourses that are associated with types and degrees of severe mental illness in the context of community-based care, discourses of "otherness", "ability", "intelligence" etc. Ethnographic investigations within the specific communities where points of care are established could further help to uncover discourses of inclusion, communal responsibility and stigma. In Chapters 3 and 5, the focus fell solely on service providers, but these accounts will invariably change when enriched by the subjectivities of service users and their families.

A particularly promising movement in improving care for severe mental and neurological conditions is shifting from discourses of containment and stability to one of recovery. The idea of recovery moves the locus of control to that of the service user, with substantial less institutional imprinting. There are many different approaches that focus on recovery, though in general it involves a close engagement with patients on develop their own recovery plans and goals, map processes, and identify barriers and facilitators to these processes. It also relies substantially on belonging and community integration as part of the recovery process. By drawing from disability studies and a capability approach, recovery has much potential to offer to people with severe mental and neurological conditions (Hopper 2007).

Recovery as imperative very much runs against the current goals of care, especially in community settings. The primary purpose of CSOs taking care of discharged patients still seem to be one of containment, rather than any kind of holistic care mandate – this is reflected by the ways in which services are measured, monitored and evaluated. We are not aware of the existence of a standardised, widely used practice of measuring changes in well-being over time – the focus very much lies on numbers of clients. Some of the larger CSOs have regular calls from the DoH asking how much space is available, that there is a need to discharge a batch of patients with no other living options outside of the state sphere. Hospital beds needs to be opened for new waves of patients, or individuals who become entangled in a perpetual revolving door syndrome. Variations of the indicator "number housed" becomes the most important mechanism the system to continue – it is the basis of funding flows, and an indication of a CSO's value to the state and the community in broad. The commodification of severe mental illness has been made possible, to some degree at least, by focusing on indicators that do not adequately include well-being, capabilities or growth. By counting the numbers of people hospitalised, discharged, taken in by a CSO, or died, without taking into consideration that people grow, change and that their recovery might be spurred on or inhibited by their environment, we are reducing people to two-dimensional entities, which increases vulnerability to exploitation. The commodification of people with severe mental and neurological conditions are supported by a legal framework that supports public-private partnerships and collaboration, without focusing on the ultimate outcomes of individuals.

What is a minimal acceptable level of care? To not die? The bottom level of Maslow's needs hierarchy, meaning food, water and housing? Or are we aiming for something more ambitious? Something in line what Sen and Nussbaum drew our attention to, that economics needs to focus on individual capabilities perhaps? This should not be termed ambitious, but rather, as per Steven Lukes (2008), values that are incommensurable. Discourses on deinstitutionalisation often centre around housing, and this is key point in relations between the state and its non-state partners. It is important however, that housing does not become an end in itself; that regulation does not only focus on and measure the state of CSO housing arrangements (for instance, by demanding certain colours of exit signs above doors, or neon yellow strips highlighting stairs – the power of health, safety and risk containment values), but focusing on the wellbeing of beneficiaries in a holistic sense. Regulating housing arrangements is a risk avoidance strategy but does not primary promote well-being. Housing certainly should be the start, though the much more pressing concern should be community integration and participation, citizenship, recovery, and citizenship (Sylvestre, Nelson, & Aubry 2017). This would require a strengthening of state-civil society relations and the solution would unfortunately not emerge from empirical work alone but would require a radical political shift.

Mental health care is intertwined with a socioeconomic system that exhibits the worst of neoliberal tendencies, and if we cannot overturn this system completely, we should at the very least work around these tendencies in such a way that people with severe mental and neurological conditions are justly cared for. Nonetheless, this is a tall, if not impossible ideal, as Wendy Brown (2003) reminds us:

> Liberal democracy cannot be submitted to neo-liberal political governmentality and survive. There is nothing in liberal democracy's basic institutions or values – from free elections, representative democracy, and individual liberties equally distributed, to modest power-sharing or even more substantive political participation – that inherently meets the test of serving economic competitiveness or inherently withstands a cost-benefit analysis.

This is an era where relationships between people are weakened, where coordinated action is devalued, where difference is flattened and inequalities obscured; resistance to these arrangements requires reclaiming the connections and spaces that are eroded by individualist values and cost effectiveness (Asen 2017). The vast body of work on mental health system strengthening, on micro, meso and macro levels of improvement, underlines the saliency of relationships and community. This realisation has emerged yet again in global health circles, with the push for people-centred, community driven health care as a democratising strategy (Martineau 2016; Sturmberg & Njoroge 2017), an approach that both serves individual outcomes and ubuntu values.

Ultimately, our task is to continue delivering work and critique aiming to improve the system of care, not because of costs containment or professional ethics, but rather because of the moral imperatives set by a just, democratic society – failure to do so would mean a triumph of Homo Economicus over Homo Sacer. A critical next step in developing this work further would be to describe the moral work of South African mental health care as an institution, which will need to entail an empirical accounting for the moral economies and moral subjectivities of mental health care. Here, moral economy means "the manner in which this issue [mental health care] is constituted through judgments and sentiments that gradually come to define a sort of common sense and collective understanding of the problem", while moral subjectivity refers to the engagement of actors with ethical sense-making in relation to each other and the system (Fassin 2015, 11). Scandals such as Life Esidimeni should not be chalked down too quickly to political manoeuvring or miscalculation without due consideration of institutional propriety or impropriety (Brown 2003), and we need to acknowledge that the institution of mental health care is, at the moment, immoral. Importantly, we need to acknowledge the limitations in merely describing power relations in Foucauldian terms. While helpful, this is but a first step, and for resistance and change to take its full form there is a need to complement descriptive practices with a normative lens, and Rawlsian insights on justice are potentially valuable here (Patton 2014).

Much in step with the blueprint set by the TRC, the achievement of social justice for people with severe mental and neurological conditions are framed by the discourse of reconciliation that naturalises subjects and objects in the political sphere, driven by secondary narratives of death and suffering (Moon 2006). Posthumous analyses – especially state-driven discourses – did not attempt to expose systematic and structural dimensions of suffering beyond the subjectivities of victims (which, one could further argue, are not true subjectivities because they were relayed by others, all of whom did not possess the subjective experience of severe mental and neurological conditions). It re-enforces the notion that victimhood is portrayed by suffering on an individual level, experienced by discrete bodies (Bowsher 2020), where in reality we can refer to a collective suffering. Borrowing Mbembe's (2019) portrayal of the slave condition in late modernity, we can describe the life of severe mental and neurological conditions as "a triple loss"; there is the loss of a home (not just physical), the loss of sovereignty over one's body, and a loss over political status. Suffering this triple loss results in the collective of people with severe mental and neurological conditions being faced with "absolute domination, natal alienation, and social death (expulsion from humanity altogether)" (p. 75).

Postscript

During the time of writing, South Africa was under a national lock down as part of the response to the arrival of the COVID-19 pandemic in the country. This was a radical move by the government, engineered to buy time, and perhaps, to take a well-needed breath in a world that is changing extremely rapidly. COVID-19 dramatically illustrated that "modern society is characterized by power that has become truly exterritorial, no longer bound, not even slowed down, by the resistance of space" (Bauman 2000, 11), a period where, as people like David Harvey (1989), Arthur Kleinman (1998) and Achille Mbembe (2019) reminds us, time-space compression has rendered us unable to cope with the sheer speed of change. To state that health systems are in a state of uncertainty is a massive understatement – there will certainly be a post-COVID world, where economic, social and cultural structures have been violently shaken. We are left to bleakly be reminded that, during times of crisis such as these, it is the poor, the vulnerable, and specifically those with severe mental illness, that will suffer the most. This makes a political economy perspective all the more pressing. While day-to-day misery surely will be amplified, there is a window for change, a portal offered to a different future. As Arundhati Roy (2020) pointed out: "And in the midst of this terrible despair, it offers us a chance to rethink the doomsday machine we have built for ourselves. Nothing could be worse than a return to normality".

Health systems are often analysed in isolation to the wider systems within which it is embedded: "Global health is typically agnostic about the kind of political system a country chooses to adopt. Global health and its institutions see health systems as separate—technically, socially, economically—from the political ideologies of nations. This view is not sustainable" (Horton 2020, 546). The lack of engagement with political and economic drivers of mental illness, despite acknowledging this primacy early on this the Movement (Lund 2015; Crick Lund, Alison Breen et al. 2010; Lund et al. 2011), remains a substantial barrier to change. Significant mental health system reform requires, in addition to close streamlining of useable science and action-oriented and contextually-relevant policy, a degree of "anger and fury" – mental health professionals, civil society and government needs to "rediscover their solidarity but also their raging soul" (Horton 2019, 1696).

References

Adut, A. (2012). A theory of the public sphere. *Sociological Theory, 30*(4), 238–262.

Adut, A. (2018). *Reign of Appearances: The Misery and Splendor of the Public Sphere*. Cambridge: Cambridge University Press.

Agamben, G. (1998). Homo Sacer. *Homo Sacer: Sovereign Power and Bare Life*. doi:10.1080/09697250802156067

Alliance for Health Policy and Systems Research (2015). What is the role of the non-state provider in achieving universal health coverage?, 24 February. Retrieved from www.who.int/alliance-hpsr/news/2015/nonstate/en/ (accessed 20 May 2020).

American Psychiatric Association (APA) (1979). Report of the committee to visit South Africa. *American Journal of Psychiatry, 136*(11), 1498–1506.

American Psychiatric Association (2013). *Diagnostic and Statistical Manual of Mental Disorders*. 5th ed. Arlington: American Psychiatric Publishing.

Androff, D. K. (2009). Truth and reconciliation commissions (TRCs): An international human rights intervention and its connection to social work. *The British Journal of Social Work, 40*(6), 1960–1977. doi:10.1093/bjsw/bcp139

Asen, R. (2017). Neoliberalism, the public sphere, and a public good. *Quarterly Journal of Speech, 103*(4), 329–349. doi:10.1080/00335630.2017.1360507

Ashmore, J. (2013). "Going private": A qualitative comparison of medical specialists' job satisfaction in the public and private sectors of South Africa. *Human Resources for Health, 11*(1), 1. doi:10.1186/1478-4491-11-1

Auchter, J. (2019). "Death in this country is normal": Quiet deaths in the Global South. In C. Alphin & F. Debrix (Eds.), *Necrogeopolitics: On Death and Death-Making in International Relations* (pp. 104–120). London: Routledge.

Axelsson, R., & Axelsson, S. B. (2006). Integration and collaboration in public health – a conceptual framework. *The International Journal of Health Planning and Management, 21*, 75–88. doi:http://dx.doi.org/10.1002/hpm.826

Bacchi, C. (2010). Foucault, policy and rule: Challenging the problem-solving paradigm. *FREIA – Feminist Research Center in Aalborg*, 1–25. doi:10.5278/freia.33190049

Batley, R. (2006). Engaged or divorced? Cross-service findings on government relations with non-state service-providers. *Public Administration and Development, 26*, 241–251.

Bauman, Z. (2000). *Liquid Modernity*. London: Wiley-Blackwell.

Binkley, S. (2011). Happiness, positive psychology and the program of neoliberal governmentality. *Subjectivity, 4*, 371–394. doi:10.1057/sub.2011.16

Birdsall, K., & Kelly, K. (2007). *Pioneers, Partners, Providers: The Dynamics of Civil Society and AIDS Funding in Southern Africa*. Johannesburg: CADRE/OSISA.

Blanchet, K., & James, P. (2012). How to do (or not to do) … a social network analysis in health systems research. *Health Policy and Planning, 27*, 438–446. doi:10.1093/heapol/czr055

Blumenfeld, J. (1997). From icon to scapegoat: The experience of South Africa's reconstruction and development programme. *Development Policy Review, 15*, 65–91.

Bond, P. (2005). *Elite Transition: From Apartheid to Neoliberalism in South Africa*. London: Pluto Press.

Bond, P. (2014). "Talk left, walk right" in South African social policy: Tokenistic extension of state welfare versus bottom-up commoning of services, University of KwaZulu-Natal School of Built Environment and Development Studies Seminar, Durban. Retrieved from http://sds.ukzn.ac.za/files/2014-02-19%20bond%20sa%20social%20policy.pdf (accessed 12 January 2017).

Borinstein, A. B. (1992). Public attitudes toward persons with mental illness. *Health Affairs, 11*(3), 186–196. doi:10.1377/hlthaff.11.3.186

Botha, U.., Koen, L., Galal, U., Jordaan, E., & Niehaus, D. J. H. (2014). The rise of assertive community interventions in South Africa: A randomized control trial assessing the impact of a modified assertive intervention on readmission rates; a three year follow-up. *BMC psychiatry, 14*, 56. doi:10.1186/1471-244X-14-56

Boucher, S., Pare, N., Perry, J. C., Sigal, J. J., & Ouimet, M. C. (2008). Consequences of an institutionalized childhood: The case of the "Duplessis orphans". *Sante Ment Que, 33*(2), 271–291. doi:10.7202/019678ar

Bourdieu, P. (1994). Rethinking the state: Genesis and structure of the bureaucratic field. *Sociological Theory, 1–18*, 1.

Bovaird, T. (2014). Efficiency in third sector partnerships for delivering local government services: The role of economies of scale, scope and learning. *Public Management Review, 16*, 1067–1090. doi:10.1080/14719037.2014.930508

Bowsher, J. (2020). The South African TRC as neoliberal reconciliation: Victim subjectivities and the synchronization of affects. *Social & Legal Studies, 29*(1), 41–64. doi:10.1177/0964663918822139

Boyd, J., & Kerr, T. (2016). Policing "Vancouver's mental health crisis": A critical discourse analysis. *Critical Public Health, 26*(4), 418–433. doi:10.1080/09581596.2015.1007923

Brazil, K., Ozer, E., Cloutier, M. M., Levine, R., Stryer, D., Lenfant, C., … Easton, S. (2005). From theory to practice: Improving the impact of health services research. *BMC Health Services Research, 5*, 1. doi:10.1186/1472-6963-5-1

Brown, W. (2003). Neo-liberalism and the end of liberal democracy. *Theory & Event, 7*(1).

Browne, G., Roberts, J., Gafni, A., Byrne, C., Kertyzia, J., & Loney, P. (2004). Conceptualizing and validating the human services integration measure. *International Journal of Integrated Care, 4*, e03.

Bruynooghe, K., Verhaeghe, M., & Bracke, P. (2008). Similarity or dissimilarity in the relations between human service organizations. *Social work in public health, 23*, 13–39. doi:10.1080/19371910802053166

Burns, J. K. (2008). Implementation of the Mental Health Care Act (2002) at district hospitals in South Africa: Translating principles into practice. *SAMJ: South African Medical Journal, 98*, 46–49.

Burstow, B. (2015). *Psychiatry and the Business of Madness: An Ethical and Epistemological Accounting*. Basingstoke: Palgrave Macmillan.

Butler, M., Kane, R., McAlpine, D., Kathol, R., Fu, S., Hagedorn, H., & Wilt, T. (2008). *Integration of Mental Health/Substance Abuse and Primary Care*, Rockville: Agency for Health care Research and Quality.

Butler, M., Kane, R., McAlpine, D., Kathol, R., Fu, S., Hagedorn, H., & Wilt, T. (2011). Does integrated care improve treatment for depression? A systematic review. *The Journal of Ambulatory Care Management, 34*, 113–125. doi:10.1097/JAC.0b013e31820ef605

Bynum, H. (2012). *Spitting Blood: The History of Tuberculosis*. Oxford: Oxford University Press.

Cammett, M. C., & MacLean, L. M. (2011). Introduction: The political consequences of non-state social welfare in the Global South. *Studies in Comparative International Development, 46*, 1–21. doi:10.1007/s12116-010-9083-7

Campbell-Hall, V., Petersen, I., Bhana, A., Mjadu, S., Hosegood, V., Flisher, A., & Consortium, T. M. R. P. (2010). Collaboration between traditional practitioners and primary health care staff in South Africa: Developing a workable partnership for community mental health services. *Transcultural Psychiatry, 47*, 610–628. doi:10.1177/1363461510383459

Carvalho, S. R. (2015). Governamentality, "liberal advanced society" and health: Dialogues with Nikolas Rose (Part 1). *Interface – Comunicação, Saúde, Educação, 19*, 647–658. doi:10.1590/1807-57622015.0216

Charlson, F. J., Baxter, A. J., Dua, T., Degenhardt, L., Whiteford, H. A., & Vos, T. (2016). Excess mortality from mental, neurological, and substance use disorders in the global burden of disease study 2010. In V. Patel, D. Chisholm, T. Dua, R. Laxminarayan, & M. E. Medina-Mora (Eds.), *Mental, Neurological, and Substance Use Disorders: Disease Control Priorities, Third Edition (Volume 4)*. Washington, DC: The International Bank for Reconstruction and Development/The World Bank.

Chatterjee, P. (2004). The politics of the governed. *The Politics of the Governed: Reflections on Popular Politics in Most of the World*, New York: Columbia University Press.

Chigwedere, P., Seage, G. R., 3rd, Gruskin, S., Lee, T. H., & Essex, M. (2008). Estimating the lost benefits of antiretroviral drug use in South Africa. *Journal of Acquired Immune Deficiency Syndromes, 49*(4), 410–415. doi:10.1097/qai.0b013e31818a6cd5

Churchyard, G., Fielding, K., Lewis, J., Coetzee, L., Godfrey-Faussett, P., & Hayes, R. (2014). A trial of communitywide isoniazid preventive therapy for tuberculosis control. *New England Journal of Medicine, 370*, 301–310.

Clark, J. N. (2012). Reconciliation via truth? A study of South Africa's TRC. *Journal of Human Rights, 11*(2), 189–209. doi:10.1080/14754835.2012.674455

Coleborne, C., & Smith, M. (2020). It's good to talk openly about mental health. Palgrave Macmillan Author Q&A. Retrieved from www.palgrave.com/gp/blogs/humanities/cathy-coleborne-and-matthew-smith (accessed 12 Jun 2020).

Collins, P. Y., Patel, V., Joestl, S. S., March, D., Insel, T. R., & Daar, A. S. (2011). Grand challenges in global mental health. *Nature, 475*, 27–30. doi:10.1038/475027a

Community Agency for Social Enquiry, Planact, & Africa Skills Development. (2008). *Review of the State of Civil Society Organisations in South Africa*. Braamfontein: National Development Agency.

Comrie, S. (2016, 11 January). Without ID, without family. *City Press*. Retrieved from https://city-press.news24.com/News/without-id-without-family-20160109 (accessed 12 February 2020).

Coovadia, H., Jewkes, R., Barron, P., Sanders, D., & McIntyre, D. (2009). The health and health system of South Africa: Historical roots of current public health challenges. *The Lancet, 374*, 817–834. doi:10.1016/S0140-6736(09)60951-X
Cornerstone Economic Research. (2018). *Performance and expenditure review: Cost implications of funding NPOs following the NAWONGO court judgements*. Research commissioned by the Government Technical Advisory Centre, National Treasury. Retrieved from: www.gtac.gov.za/Pages/PER_Nawongo-Implications (accessed 18 November 2019).
Cosgrove, L., & Karter, J. M. (2018). The poison in the cure: Neoliberalism and contemporary movements in mental health. *Theory & Psychology, 28*(5), 669–683. doi:10.1177/0959354318796307
Craven, M., & Bland, R. (2006). Better practices in collaborative mental health care: An analysis of the evidence base. *Canadian Journal of Psychiatry, 51*, 7s–72s.
Cresswell, J. W. (2014). *Research Design: Qualitative, Quantitative and Mixed Methods Approaches.* Los Angeles: SAGE Publications.
Cristofoli, D., Meneguzzo, M., & Riccucci, N. (2017). Collaborative administration: the management of successful networks. *Public Management Review, 19*, 275–283. doi:10.1080/14719037.2016.1209236
D'Amour, D., Goulet, L., Labadie, J.-f., Martín-Rodriguez, L. S., & Pineault, R. (2008). A model and typology of collaboration between professionals in health care organizations. *14*, 1–14. doi:10.1186/1472-6963-8-188
de Mooij, L. D., Kikkert, M., Theunissen, J., Beekman, A. T. F., de Haan, L., Duurkoop, P. W. R. A., … Dekker, J. J. M. (2019). Dying too soon: Excess mortality in severe mental illness. *Frontiers in Psychiatry, 10*, 855-855. doi:10.3389/fpsyt.2019.00855
de Villiers, F. (1975, 27 April). Millions out of madness. *Sunday Times*.
Deleuze, G. (2004) *Desert Islands and Other Texts 1953–1974*. Edited by D. Lapoujade. New York: Semiotext(e).
Development Bank of Southern Africa. (2008). *A Roadmap for the Reform of the South African Health System*. Midrand: DBSA.
Devereux, S., & Solomon, C. (2011). Can social protection deliver social justice for farmwomen in South Africa? In *International Conference: Social Protection for Social Justice*. Brighton: Institute of Development Studies, University of Sussex.
Dickinson, H., & Glasby, J. (2010). "Why partnership working doesn't work". *Public Management Review, 12*, 811–828. doi:10.1080/14719037.2010.488861
Docrat, S., Besada, D., Cleary, S., Daviaud, E., & Lund, C. (2019). Mental health system costs, resources and constraints in South Africa: A national survey. *Health Policy and Planning, 34*(9), 706–719. doi:10.1093/heapol/czz085
Docrat, S., Lund, C., & Besada, D. (2019). *An Evaluation of the Health System Costs of Mental Health Services and Programmes in South Africa*. Cape Town: Alan J Flisher Centre for Public Mental Health & the South African Medical Research Council.
Donahue, J. (2004). *On Collaborative Governance.* Corporate Social Responsibility Initiative Working Paper No. 2, Cambridge, MA.
Doolin, B. (2004). Power and resistance in the implementation of a medical management information system. *Information Systems Journal, 14*, 343–362.
Draper, C. E., Lund, C., Kleintjes, S., Funk, M., Omar, M., Flisher, A. J., … Petersen, I. (2009). Mental health policy in South Africa: Development process and content. *Health Policy and Planning, 24*, 342–356. doi:10.1093/heapol/czp027

Du Toit, M. (1996). *Women, welfare and the nurturing of Afrikaner nationalism: A social history of the Afrikaanse Christelike Vroue Vereniging, c.1870–1939.* PhD diss., University of Cape Town. Retrieved from http://hdl.handle.net/11427/26212 (accessed 14 March 2020).

Durbin, J., Goering, P., Streiner, D. L., & Pink, G. (2006). Does systems integration affect continuity of mental health care? *Administration and Policy in Mental Health and Mental Health Services Research, 33*, 705–717. doi:10.1007/s10488-006-0087-6

Econex. (2017). *The Economic Footprint of Private Hospital Groups in South Africa: A Multiplier Study*. Report prepared for the Hospital Association of South Africa (HASA). Stellenbosch: Econex.

Eghigian, G. (2010) *From Madness to Mental Health: Psychiatric Disorder and Its Treatment in Western Civilization*. New Brunswick, NJ: Rutgers University Press.

Emerson, K., Nabatchi, T., & Balogh, S. (2012). An integrative framework for collaborative governance. *Journal of Public Administration Research and Theory, 22*, 1–29. doi:10.1093/jopart/mur011

Erasmus, E., & Gilson, L. (2008). How to start thinking about investigating power in the organizational settings of policy implementation. *Health Policy and Planning, 23*, 361–368. doi:10.1093/heapol/czn021

Evans, B. C., Coon, D. W., & Ume, E. (2011). Use of theoretical frameworks as a pragmatic guide for mixed methods studies: A methodological necessity? *Journal of Mixed Methods Research, 5*, 276–292. doi:10.1177/1558689811412972

Farham, B. (2017). Cry, the beloved country. *SAMJ: South African Medical Journal, 107*, 277–277.

Fassin, D. (2015). Can states be moral? In D. Fassin (Ed.), *At the Heart of the State: The Moral World of Institutions* (pp. i–xi). London: Pluto Press.

Fedderke, J. (2009). *Social welfare: Social stasis*. Helen Suzman Foundation. Retrieved from https://hsf.org.za/publications/focus/focus-55-november-2009-images-of-justice/social-welfare-social-stasis/view (accessed 15 March 2020).

Ferguson, J. (2006). *Global Shadows: Africa in the Neoliberal World Order*. Durham, NC: Duke University Press.

Ferguson, J. (2015). *Give a Man a Fish: Reflections on the New Politics of Distribution*. Durham, NC: Duke University Press.

Fimreite, A. L., & Lægreid, P. (2009). Reorganizing the welfare state administration: Partnership, networks and accountability. *Public Management Review, 11*, 281–297. doi:10.1080/14719030902798198

Fine, B., & Saad-Filho, A. (2017). Thirteen things you need to know about neoliberalism. *Critical Sociology, 43*(4–5), 685–706. doi:10.1177/0896920516655387

Fleury, M.-J. (2005). Quebec mental health services networks: Models and implementation. *International Journal of Integrated Care, 5*, 1.

Fleury, M.-J., Grenier, G., Bamvita, J.-M., Wallot, H., & Michel, P. (2012). Determinants of referral to the public health care and social sector by nonprofit organizations: Clinical profile and interorganizational characteristics. *Nonprofit and Voluntary Sector Quarterly, 41*, 257–279.

Fleury, M., Mercier, C., & Denis, J.-L. (2002). Regional planning implementation and its impact on integration of a mental health care network. *International Journal of Health Planning {&} Management, 17*, 315–332. doi:10.1002/hpm.684

Fleury, M. J., Grenier, G., Vallee, C., Aube, D., Farand, L., Bamvita, J. M., & Cyr, G. (2016). Implementation of the Quebec mental health reform (2005–2015). *BMC Health Services Research, 16*(1), 586. doi:10.1186/s12913-016-1832-5

Foucault, M. (1978). *The History of Sexuality Volume 1: An Introduction* (R. Hurley, Trans.). New York: Random House.

Foucault, M. (2008) *The Birth of Biopolitics: Lectures at the College de France 1978–1979*. Basingstoke: Palgrave Macmillan.

Fountoulakis, K. N., & Möller, H.-J. (2011). Efficacy of antidepressants: A re-analysis and re-interpretation of the Kirsch data. *International Journal of Neuropsychopharmacology, 14*(3), 405–412. doi:10.1017/s1461145710000957

Fourie, J., & Gagiano, C. A. (1988). A modern community psychiatric service in the Orange Free State. *South African Medical Journal, 73*(7), 427–429.

Fourie, P. (2006). *The Political Management of HIV and AIDS in South Africa: One Burden Too Many?* Basingstoke: Palgrave Macmillan.

Free State High Court (2010). *National Association of Welfare Organisations and Non-Governmental Organisations and Others v Member of the Executive Council for Social Development, Free State and Others (1719/2010) ZAFSHC 127, Southern African Legal Information Institute.* Retrieved from www.saflii.org/za/cases/ZAFSHC/2010/127.html (accessed 18 November 2015).

Free State High Court (2011). *National Association of Welfare Organisations and Non-Governmental Organisations and Others v Member of the Executive Council for Social Development, Free State and Others (1719/2010) ZAFSHC 127, Southern African Legal Information Institute.* Retrieved from www.saflii.info/za/cases/ZAFSHC/2011/84.html (accessed 18 November 2015).

Free State High Court (2014). *National Association of Welfare Organisations and Non-Governmental Organisations and Others v Member of the Executive Council for Social Development, Free State and Others (1719/2010) [2014] ZAFSHC 127, Southern African Legal Information Institute*. Retrieved from www.saflii.org/za/cases/ZAFSHC/2014/127.html (accessed 18 November 2015).

Frenk, J., & Moon, S. (2013). Governance challenges in global health. *New England Journal of Medicine, 368*, 936–942. doi:10.1056/NEJMra1109339

Fuller, D. A., Lamb, H. R., Biasotti, M., & Snook, J. (2015). *Overlooked in the undercounted: The role of mental illness in fatal law enforcement encounters*. Arlington, VA: Office of Research and Public Affairs.

Gillis, L. (2012) The historical development of psychiatry in South Africa since 1652. *South African Journal of Psychiatry*, *18*(3), p. 78. doi: 10.7196/SAJP.355.

Gilson, L. (2007). *What Sort of Stewardship and Health System Management Is Needed To Tackle Health Inequity, and How Can It Be Developed and Sustained? A Literature Review*. London: Knowledge Network on Health Systems, of the Commission on the Social Determinants of Health.

Gilson, L., & Daire, J. (2011). Leadership and governance within the South African health system. *South African Health Review*, 69–80.

Gilson, L., & Raphaely, N. (2008). The terrain of health policy analysis in low and middle income countries: A review of published literature 1994–2007. *Health Policy and Planning, 23*, 294–307. doi:10.1093/heapol/czn019

Gitlin, M. J., & Miklowitz, D. J. (2014). Psychiatric diagnosis in ICD-11: Lessons learned (or not) from the mood disorders section in DSM-5. *Australian and New Zealand Journal of Psychiatry, 48*(1), 89–90. doi:10.1177/0004867413515952

Glendinning, C. (2003). Breaking down barriers: Integrating health and care services for older people in England. *Health Policy, 65*, 139–151. doi:10.1016/S0168-8510(02)00205-1

Goldman, H. H., & Morrissey, J. P. (1985). The alchemy of mental health policy: Homelessness and the fourth cycle of reform. *American Journal of Public Health, 75*(7), 727–731.

Goldman, H. H. and Grob, G. N. (2006) Defining "mental illness" in mental health policy. *Health Affairs, 25*(3). doi: 10.1377/hlthaff.25.3.737.

Goodwin, N. (2010). It's good to talk: Social network analysis as a method for judging the strength of integrated care. *International Journal of Integrated Care, 10*, 1–2.

Government Technical Advisory Centre. (2018). Cost implications of the NAWONGO court judgements. Retrieved from www.gtac.gov.za/perdetail/Infographics.pdf (accessed 23 January 2020).

Groopman, J. (2019, 27 May). The Troubled History of Psychiatry. *The New Yorker*. Retrieved from www.newyorker.com/magazine/2019/05/27/the-troubled-history-of-psychiatry (accessed 12 December 2019).

Habermas, J. (1991). *The Structural Transformation of the Public Sphere: An Inquiry into a Category of Bourgeois Society* (T. Burger & F. Lawrence Eds.). Cambridge, MA: MIT Press.

Habermas, J. (1995). Reconciliation through the public use of reason: Remarks on John Rawls's political liberalism. *The Journal of Philosophy, 92*(3), 109–131. doi:10.2307/2940842

Habib, A. (2005). State-civil society relations in post-apartheid South Africa. *Social Research, 72*, 671–692.

Habib, A., & Taylor, R. (1999). South Africa: Anti-Apartheid NGOs in transition. In *Voluntas: International Journal of Voluntary and Nonprofit Organizations, 10*, 73–82.

Hacking, I. (2013) Lost in the forest. *London Review of Books, 35*(15), 7–8.

Halpern, J., & Weinstein, H. M. (2004). Empathy and rehumanization after mass violence. In E. Stover & H. M. Weinstein (Eds.), *My Neighbor, My Enemy: Justice and Community in the Aftermath of Mass Atrocity* (pp. 303–322). Cambridge: Cambridge University Press.

Hanlon, C., Eshetu, T., Alemayedu, D., Fekadu, A., Semrau, M., Thornicroft, G., … Alem, A. (2017). Health system governance to support the scale up of mental health care in Ethiopia: a qualitative study. *International Journal of Mental Health Systems, 11*. doi:10.1186/s13033-017-0144-4

Hanlon, C., Luitel, N. P., Kathree, T., Murhar, V., Shrivasta, S., Medhin, G., … Prince, M. (2014). Challenges and opportunities for implementing integrated mental health care: A district level situation analysis from five low- and middle-income countries. *PLOS ONE, 9*. doi:10.1371/journal.pone.0088437

Hannigan, B., & Coffey, M. (2011). Where the wicked problems are: The case of mental health. *Health Policy, 101*, 220–227. doi:10.1016/j.healthpol.2010.11.002

Harcourt, B. (2011). *The Punitive Order: Free Markets, Neoliberalism, and Mass Incarceration in the United States*. Paper presented at the Reflecting on 20 years of The Foucault Effect: Studies in Governmentality, Birkbeck College, University of London. https://backdoorbroadcasting.net/2011/06/jonathan-simon-from-the-medical-model-to-the-humanitarian-crisis-model-californias-prison-health-crisis-and-the-future-of-imprisonment/ (accessed 23 November 2019).

Harcourt, B. (2015). Mass incarceration in the USA. *Michel Foucault's College de France Lectures*. Retrieved from http://blogs.law.columbia.edu/foucault1313/2015/10/25/foucault-313-the-punitive-society-mass-incarceration-in-the-usa/ (accessed 23 November 2019).

Harris, B., Eyles, J., & Goudge, J. (2016). Ways of doing: Restorative practices, governmentality, and provider conduct in post-apartheid health care. *Medical Anthropology, 9740*, 1–17. doi:10.1080/01459740.2016.1173691

Harris, B., Goudge, J., Ataguba, J. E., McIntyre, D., Nxumalo, N., Jikwana, S., & Chersich, M. (2011). Inequities in access to health care in South Africa. *Journal of Public Health Policy, 32*, S102-S123. doi:10.1057/jphp.2011.35

Harrison, D. (2009). An overview of health and health care in South Africa 1994–2010: Priorities, progress and prospects for new gains. *A Discussion Document Commissioned by the Henry J Kaiser Family Foundation to Help Inform the National Health Leaders' Retreat Muldersdrift*, 1–40.

Hart, G. (2008). The provocations of neoliberalism: Contesting the nation and liberation after apartheid. *Antipode, 40*(4), 678–705. doi:10.1111/j.1467-8330.2008.00629.x

Hart, G. (2012). Replacing the nation: South Africa's passive revolution? Public lecture, London School of Economics, Tuesday 4 December.

Hart, G. (2013) *Rethinking the South African Crisis: Nationalism, Populism, Hegenomy*. Durban: University of KwaZulu-Natal Press.

Hart, G. (2015). Political society and its discontents. *Economic and Political Weekly, 50*(43), 43–51.

Harvey, D. (1989). *The Condition of Postmodernity: An Enquiry into the Origins of Cultural Change*. Oxford: Blackwell Publishers.

Harvey, D. (2005) *A Brief History of Neoliberalism*. Oxford: Oxford University Press.

Heen, H. (2009). One size does not fit all. *Public Management Review, 11*, 235–253. doi:10.1080/14719030802685263

Heinrich, V. F. (2001). The role of NGOs in strengthening the foundations of South African democracy. *Voluntas: International Journal of Voluntary and Nonprofit Organizations, 12*(1), 1–15. doi:10.1023/A:1011217326747

Hidaka, B. H. (2012). Depression as a disease of modernity: Explanations for increasing prevalence. *Journal of Affective Disorders, 140*(3), 205–214. doi:10.1016/j.jad.2011.12.036

Hill, C., & Lynn, L. (2003). Producing human services: Why do agencies collaborate? *Public Management Review, 5*, 63–81. doi:10.1080/1461667022000028861

Hochschild, A. (2014, 6 March). *Object of Plunder: The Congo through the Centuries.* Paper presented at the Connecting Seas: A Visual History of Discoveries and Encounters, Getty Research Institute. Retrieved from www.youtube.com/watch?v=rLyZGTwmcRA (accessed 23 April 2020).

Holmes, D., & Gastaldo, D. (2002). Nursing as means of governmentality. *Journal of Advanced Nursing, 38*, 557–565. doi:10.1046/j.1365-2648.2002.02222.x

Hopper, K. (2007). Rethinking social recovery in schizophrenia: What a capabilities approach might offer. *Social Science & Medicine, 65*(5), 868–879. doi:10.1016/j.socscimed.2007.04.012

Horton, R. (2007). Launching a new movement for mental health. *Lancet, 370*, 806. doi:10.1016/S0140-6736(07)61243-4

Horton, R. (2019). Offline: A perilous birthday party for mental health. *Lancet, 394*(10210), 1696. doi:10.1016/s0140-6736(19)32716-3

Horton, R. (2020). Offline: Facts are not enough. *Lancet, 395*(10224), 546. doi:10.1016/s0140-6736(20)30405-0

Hultberg, E., Lonnroth, K., & Allebeck, P. (2005). Interdisciplinary collaboration between primary care, social insurance and social services in the rehabilitation of people with musculoskeletal disorder: Effects on self-related health and physical performance. *Journal of Interprofessional Care, 19*, 115–124.

Hunter, D., & Perkins, N. (2012). Partnership working in public health: The implications for governance of a systems approach. *Journal of Health Services Research & Policy, 17*, 45–52. doi:10.1258/jhsrp.2012.011127

Ikkos, G., Boardman, J., & Zigmond, T. (2006). Talking liberties: John Rawls's theory of justice and psychiatric practice. *Advances in Psychiatric Treatment, 12*(3), 202–210. doi:10.1192/apt.12.3.202

International Labour Organization (2013). *The Potential of Non-Profit Organizations in the Free State Province to Adopt a Social Enterprise Approach* Geneva: ILO.

Jack, H., Wagner G., R. G., Petersen, I., Thom, R., Newton R., C. R., Stein, A., … Hofman, K. J. (2014). Closing the mental health treatment gap in South Africa: A review of costs and cost-effectiveness. *Global Health Action, 7*. doi:10.3402/gha.v7.23431

Jakobsen, J. C., Katakam, K. K., Schou, A., Hellmuth, S. G., Stallknecht, S. E., Leth-Møller, K., … Gluud, C. (2017). Selective serotonin reuptake inhibitors versus placebo in patients with major depressive disorder: A systematic review with meta-analysis and trial sequential analysis. *BMC Psychiatry, 17*(1), 58. doi:10.1186/s12888-016-1173-2

Janse van Rensburg, A. (2018). *Governance and Power in Mental Health Integration Processes in South Africa.* (PhD). Ghent University and Stellenbosch University, Ghent, Belgium/Stelenbosch, South Africa.

Janse van Rensburg, A., & Fourie, P. (2016). Health policy and integrated mental health care in the SADC region: Strategic clarification using the Rainbow Model. *International Journal of Mental Health Systems*, 1–13. doi:10.1186/s13033-016-0081-7

Janse van Rensburg, A., Khan, R., Wouters, E., van Rensburg, D., Fourie, P., & Bracke, P. (2018). At the coalface of collaborative mental health care: A qualitative study of governance and power in district-level service provision in South Africa. *International Journal of Health Planning and Management, 33*. doi:10.1002/hpm.2593

Janse van Rensburg, A., Petersen, I., Wouters, E., Engelbrecht, M., Kigozi, G., Fourie, P., … Bracke, P. (2018). State and non-state mental health service collaboration in a South African district: A mixed methods study. *Health Policy Plan, 33*(4), 516–527. doi:10.1093/heapol/czy017

Janse van Rensburg, A., Rau, A., Fourie, P., & Bracke, P. (2016). Power and integrated health care: Shifting from governance to governmentality. *International Journal of Integrated Care, 16*, 1–11.

Janse van Rensburg, A., Wouters, E., Fourie, P., van Rensburg, D., & Bracke, P. (2018). Collaborative mental health care in the bureaucratic field of post-apartheid South Africa. *Health Sociology Review, 27*(3), 279–293. doi:10.1080/14461242.2018.14796510

Janse van Rensburg, B. (2011). Available resources and human rights: A South African perspective. *African Journal of Psychiatry, 14*, 173–175.

Janse van Rensburg, B. (2017). Life Esidimeni psychiatric patients in Gauteng Province, South Africa: clinicians' voices and activism – an ongoing, but submerged narrative. *South African Journal of Bioethics and Law, 10*(2), 44–47. doi: http://dx.doi.org/10.7196/SAJBL.2017.v10i2.614

Jessop, B. (2016). *The State: Past, Present, Future*. Cambridge: Polity Press.

Jewkes, R. (1984). *The Case for South Africa's Explusion from International Psychiatry*. New York: UN Centre against Apartheid.

John, A., McGregor, J., Jones, I., Lee, S. C., Walters, J. T. R., Owen, M. J., … Lloyd, K. (2018). Premature mortality among people with severe mental illness – New evidence from linked primary care data. *Schizophrenia Research, 199*, 154–162. doi:https://doi.org/10.1016/j.schres.2018.04.009

Johnson, R. B., & Onwuegbuzie, A. J. (2004). Mixed methods research: A research paradigm whose time has come. *Educational Researcher, 33*, 14–26.

Jones, T. F. (2012). *Psychiatry, Mental Institutions, and the Mad in Apartheid South Africa.* New York: Routledge.

Kahneman, D. (2011). *Thinking, Fast and Slow*. New York: Macmillan.

Karriem, A., & Hoskins, M. (2016). From the RDP to the NDP: A critical appraisal of the developmental state, land reform, and rural development in South Africa. *Politikon, 43*, 325–343. doi:10.1080/02589346.2016.1160858

Khan, A., & Brown, W. A. (2015). Antidepressants versus placebo in major depression: An overview. *World Psychiatry: Official Journal of the World Psychiatric Association (WPA), 14*(3), 294–300. doi:10.1002/wps.20241

Khan, A., Fahl Mar, K., Faucett, J., Khan Schilling, S., & Brown, W. A. (2017). Has the rising placebo response impacted antidepressant clinical trial outcome? Data from the US Food and Drug Administration 1987–2013. *World Psychiatry, 16*(2), 181–192. doi:10.1002/wps.20421

Kirsch, I. (2011). *The Emperor's New Drugs: Exploding the Antidepressant Myth.* New York: Basic Books.

Kirsch, I. (2019). Placebo effect in the treatment of depression and anxiety. *Frontiers in Psychiatry, 10*(407). doi:10.3389/fpsyt.2019.00407

Kirsch, I., Deacon, B. J., Huedo-Medina, T. B., Scoboria, A., Moore, T. J., & Johnson, B. T. (2008). Initial severity and antidepressant benefits: A meta-analysis of data submitted to the Food and Drug Administration. *PLOS Medicine, 5*(2), e45. doi:10.1371/journal.pmed.0050045

Kleinman, A. (1998) Experience and its moral modes: Culture, human conditions and disorder. In G. B. Peterson (Ed.), *The Tanner Lectures on Human Values* (Vol. 20, pp. 357–420). Salt Lake City: University of Utah Press.

Kleinman, A., Estrin, G. L., Usmani, S., Chisholm, D., Marquez, P. V., Evans, T. G., & Saxena, S. (2016). Time for mental health to come out of the shadows. *The Lancet, 387*, 2274–2275. doi:10.1016/S0140-6736(16)30655-9

Kodner, D. L. (2009). All together now: A conceptual exploration of integrated care. *Health care Quarterly, 13*, 6–15. doi:doi:10.12927/hcq.2009.21091

Kodner, D. L., & Spreeuwenberg, C. (2002). Integrated care: Meaning, logic, applications, and implications – a discussion paper. *International Journal of Integrated Care, 2*, e12. doi:ISSN 1568–4156

Konieczna, A., & Skinner, R. (2019). *A Global History of Anti-Apartheid: "Forward to Freedom" in South Africa*. London: Palgrave Macmillan.

Koyanagi, C. (2007). *Learning from History: Deinstitutionalization of People with Mental Illness as Precursor to Long-Term Care Reform.* Retrieved from www.kff.org/wp-content/uploads/2013/01/7684.pdf (accessed 13 November 2020).

Krüger, C., & Lewis, C. (2011). Patient and social work factors related to successful placement of long-term psychiatric in-patients from a specialist psychiatric hospital in South Africa. *African Journal of Psychiatry, 14*, 120–129.

The Lancet (2013). A revolution in psychiatry. *The Lancet, 381*(9881), 1878. doi:10.1016/S0140-6736(13)61143-5

Lancet Global Mental Health Group (2007). Scale up services for mental disorders: A call for action. *The Lancet, 370*(9594), 1241–1252. doi:10.1016/S0140-6736(07)61242-2

Lehmann, U., & Gilson, L. (2013). Actor interfaces and practices of power in a community health worker programme: A South African study of unintended policy outcomes. *Health Policy and Planning, 28*, 358–366. doi:10.1093/heapol/czs066

Lehmann, U., & Gilson, L. (2015). Action learning for health system governance: The reward and challenge of co-production. *Health Policy and Planning, 30*, 957–963. doi:10.1093/heapol/czu097

Lisi, L. F. (2015). Tragedy, history, and the form of philosophy in either/or. *2015, 7*, 30. doi:10.5399/uo/konturen.7.0.3673

Lorant, V., Nazroo, J., Nicaise, P., & Group, T. T. S. (2017). Optimal network for patients with severe mental illness: A social network analysis. *Administration and Policy in Mental Health and Mental Health Services Research, 44*, 877–887.

Lukes, S. (2008). *Moral Relativism.* London: Profile Books.

Lund, C. (2015). Poverty, inequality and mental health in low- and middle-income countries: Time to expand the research and policy agendas. *Epidemiology and Psychiatric Sciences, 24*, 97–99. doi:10.1017/S2045796015000050

Lund, C., Breen, A., Flisher, A. J., Kakuma, R., Corrigall, J., Joska, J. A., … Patel, V. (2010). Poverty and common mental disorders in low and middle income countries: A systematic review. *Social Science and Medicine, 71*, 517–528. doi:10.1016/j.socscimed.2010.04.027

Lund, C., De Silva, M., Plagerson, S., Cooper, S., Chisholm, D., Das, J., … Patel, V. (2011). Poverty and mental disorders: Breaking the cycle in low-income and middle-income countries. *The Lancet, 378*, 1502–1514. doi:10.1016/S0140-6736(11)60754-X

Lund, C., & Flisher, A. J. (2001). South African mental health process indicators. *Journal of Mental Health Policy and Economics, 4*(1), 9–16.

Lund, C., & Flisher, A. J. (2003). Community/hospital indicators in South African public sector mental health services. *Journal of Mental Health Policy and Economics, 6*(4), 181–187.

Lund, C., & Flisher, A. J. (2006). Norms for mental health services in South Africa. *Social Psychiatry and Psychiatric Epidemiology, 41*(7), 587–594. doi:10.1007/s00127-006-0057-z

Lund, C., & Flisher, A. J. (2009). A model for community mental health services in South Africa. *Tropical Medicine and International Health, 14*, 1040–1047. doi:10.1111/j.1365-3156.2009.02332.x

Lund, C., Flisher, A. J., Porteus, K., & Lee, T. (2002). Bed/population ratios in South African public sector mental health services. *Social Psychiatry and Psychiatric Epidemiology, 37*(7), 346–349. doi:10.1007/s00127-002-0552-9

Lund, C., Kleintjes, S., Kakuma, R., & Flisher, A. J. (2010). Public sector mental health systems in South Africa: Inter-provincial comparisons and policy implications. *Social Psychiatry and Psychiatric Epidemiology, 45*, 393–404. doi:10.1007/s00127-009-0078-5

Lund, C., Petersen, I., Kleintjes, S., & Bhana, A. (2012). Mental health services in South Africa: taking stock. *African Journal of Psychiatry (Johannesburg), 15*(6), 402–405. doi:http://dx.doi.org/10.4314/ajpsy.v15i6.48 10.4314/ajpsy.v15i6.48

Lund, C., Petersen, I., Kleintjes, S., & Bhana, A. (2012). Mental health services in South Africa: Taking stock. *Afr J Psychiatry (Johannesbg), 15*(6), 402–405.

Lund, C., Tomlinson, M., & Patel, V. (2016). Integration of mental health into primary care in low- and middle-income countries: The PRIME mental health care plans. *The British Journal of Psychiatry, 208*, s1-s3. doi:10.1192/bjp.bp.114.153668

Luo, Q., Chen, Q., Wang, W., Desrivieres, S., Quinlan, E. B., Jia, T., … Feng, J. (2019). Association of a schizophrenia-risk nonsynonymous variant with putamen volume in adolescents: A voxelwise and genome-wide association study. *JAMA Psychiatry, 76*(4), 435–445. doi:10.1001/jamapsychiatry.2018.4126

Mackintosh, M. (2013). *Health Care Commercialisation: A Core Development Issue.* Public lecture delivered on 16 May, Birkbeck, University of London. London: University of London. Retrieved from https://backdoorbroadcasting.net/2013/05/maureen-mackintosh-health-care-commercialisation-a-core-development-issue/ (accessed 12 May 2017).

Mahlangu, Q. (2015a). Gauteng Department of Health 2015–2016 Budget Speech. Pretoria: Gauteng Department of Health.

Mahlangu, Q. (2015b). South Africa: Gauteng Health Terminates Life Health care Esidimeni Contract. Pretoria: Gauteng Department of Health.

Makgoba, M. (2017). *Report into the Circumstances Surrounding the Deaths of Mentally Ill Patients: Gauteng Province*. Pretoria: Office of Health Standards Compliance.

Mann, M. (1993). *The Sources of Social Power Vol 2: The Rise of Classes and Nation-states, 1760–1914.* Cambridge: Cambridge University Press.

Maphanga, C. (2018, 12 December). "I will only be happy when Qedani Mahlangu is in jail" – Life Esidimeni family member. *News24*. Retrieved from www.news24.com/SouthAfrica/News/i-will-only-be-happy-when-qedani-mahlangu-is-in-jail-life-esidimeni-family-member-20181212 (accessed 12 October 2019).

Maregele, B. (2017) *SASSA Withdraws Application to Constitutional Court Hours after Filing It, GroundUp*. Retrieved from www.groundup.org.za/article/sassa-withdraws-application-constitutional-court-hours-after-filing-it/ (accessed 26 October 2017).

Markovic, J. (2017). Contingencies and organizing principles in public networks. *Public Management Review, 19*, 361–380. doi:10.1080/14719037.2016.1209237

Marshall, D. J., & Staeheli, L. (2015). Mapping civil society with social network analysis: Methodological possibilities and limitations. *Geoforum, 61*, 56–66. doi:10.1016/j.geoforum.2015.02.015

Martineau, F. P. (2016). People-centred health systems: Building more resilient health systems in the wake of the Ebola crisis. *International health, 8*(5), 307–309.

Maruthappu, M., Hasan, A., & Zeltner, T. (2015). Enablers and barriers in implementing integrated care. *Health Systems & Reform, 1*, 250–256. doi:10.1080/23288604.2015.1077301

Marx, K. (1977). Results of the immediate process of production. In D. McLellan (Ed.), *Karl Marx: Selected Writings*. Oxford: Oxford University Press.

May, P. J., & Winter, S. C. (2009). Politicians, managers, and street-level bureaucrats: Influences on policy implementation. *Journal of Public Administration Research and Theory, 19*, 453–476. doi:10.1093/jopart/mum030

Mayosi, B. M., & Benatar, S. R. (2014). Health and health care in South Africa – 20 years after Mandela. *New England Journal of Medicine, 371*(14), 1344–1353. doi:10.1056/NEJMsr1405012

Mayosi, B. M., Lawn, J. E., Niekerk, A. V., Bradshaw, D., Karim, S. S. A., Coovadia, H. M., & South, L. (2012). Review health in South Africa: Changes and challenges since 2009. *www.thelancet.com, 380*, 5–19. doi:doi.org/10.1016/S0140-6736(12)61814–5

Mbembe, A. (2019). *Necropolitics*. Durham, NC: Duke University Press.

Mechanic, D. (1990). Deinstitutionalisation: An appraisal of reform. *Annual Review of Sociology, 16*, 301–327.

Mechanic, D. (1994). *Inescapable Decisions: The Imperatives of Health Reform.* New Brunswick, NJ: CC.

Mechanic, D. (2003). Policy challenges in improving mental health services: some lessons from the past. *Psychiatric Services, 54*, 1227–1232.

Mechanic, D., Mcalpine, D. D., & Rochefort, D. A. (2014). *Mental Health and Social Policy: Beyond Managed Care.* 6th ed. Boston: Pearson Education.

Microsoft Corporation (2010). Microsoft Office Professional Plus.

Mik-Meyer, N., & Silverman, D. (2019). Agency and clientship in public encounters: Co-constructing "neediness" and "worthiness" in shelter placement meetings. *The British Journal of Sociology, 70*(5), 1640–1660. doi:10.1111/1468-4446.12633

Miller, P. (2001). Governing by numbers: Why calculative practices matter. *Social Research, 68*, 379–396. doi:10.2307/40971463

Miller, P., & Rose, N. (2008). *Governing the Present: Administering Economic, Social and Personal Life.* Cambridge: Polity Press.

Millward, H. B., Provan, K. G., Fish, A., Isett, K. R., & Huang, K. (2009). Governance and collaboration: An evolutionary study of two mental health networks. *Journal of Public Administration Research and Theory, 20*, 125–141. doi:10.1093/jopart/mup038

Mitchell, S. M., & Shortell, S. M. (2000). The governance and management of effective community health partnerships: A typology for research, policy, and practice. *Milbank Quarterly, 78*, 151,241–289. doi:10.1111/1468-0009.00170

Mitlin, D., Hickey, S., & Bebbington, A. (2007). Reclaiming development? NGOs and the challenge of alternatives. *World Development, 35*, 1699–1720.

Mkhwanazi, A. (2015). Halfway between help and home. Retrieved from https://health-e.org.za/2015/01/06/halfway-help-home/ (accessed 17 October 2019).

Mkize, D. L., Green-Thompson, R. W., Ramdass, P., Mhlaluka, G., Dlamini, N., & Walker, J. (2004). Mental health services in KwaZulu-Natal. *2004, 10*(1). doi:10.4102/sajpsychiatry.v10i1.116

Mkize, L. P., & Uys, L. R. (2004). Pathways to mental health care in KwaZulu–Natal. *Curationis, 27*(3), 62–71. doi:10.4102/curationis.v27i3.1001

Mogoeng, C. et al. (2017). *Black Sash Trust v Minister of Social Development and Others* [2017] ZACC 8, Constitutional Court of South Africa.

Moncrieff, J. (2008). *The Myth of the Chemical Cure: A Critique of Psychiatric Drug Treatment.* Basingstoke: Palgrave Macmillan.

Moncrieff, J., & Kirsch, I. (2005). Efficacy of antidepressants in adults. *BMJ (Clinical Research Ed.), 331*(7509), 155–157. doi:10.1136/bmj.331.7509.155

Moncrieff, J., Wessely, S., & Hardy, R. (2004). Active placebos versus antidepressants for depression. *Cochrane Database of Systematic Review,* (1), Cd003012. doi:10.1002/14651858.CD003012.pub2

Moncrieff, J. (2014). The medicalisation of "ups and downs": The marketing of the new bipolar disorder. *Transcultural Psychiatry, 51*(4), 581–598. doi: 10.1177/1363461514530024.

Moon, C. (2006). Narrating political reconciliation: Truth and reconciliation in South Africa. *Social & Legal Studies, 15*(2), 257–275. doi:10.1177/0964663906063582

Moosa, M. Y. H., & Jeenah, F. Y. (2008). Community psychiatry: An audit of the services in southern Gauteng. *South African Journal of Psychiatry, 14*, 36–43.

Morrow, M., Dagg, P. K. B., & Pederson, A. (2008). Is deinstitutionalization a 'failed experiment'? The ethics of re-institutionalization. *Journal of Ethics in Mental Health, 3*, 1–7.

Moseneke, D. (2018). *Life Esidimeni Arbitration Award: Families of mental health care users affected by the Gauteng Mental Marathon Project (Claimants) and National Minister of Health of the Republic of South Africa.* Government of the Province of Gauteng, Premier of the Province of Gauteng, Member of the Executive Council of Health: Province of Gauteng.

Moshabela, M., Gitomer, S., Qhibi, B., & Schneider, H. (2013). Development of non-profit organisations providing health and social services in rural South Africa: A three-year longitudinal study. *PLOS ONE, 8*(12), e83861. doi:10.1371/journal.pone.0083861

Müller, M.-M. (2014). De-monopolizing the bureaucratic field. *Alternatives: Global, Local, Political, 39*, 37–54. doi:10.1177/0304375414560467

Mur-Veeman, I., Hardy, B., Steenbergen, M., & Wistow, G. (2003). Development of integrated care in England and the Netherlands: Managing across public-private boundaries. *Health Policy, 65*, 227–241. doi:10.1016/S0168-8510(02)00215-4

Mur-Veeman, I., Van Raak, A., & Paulus, A. (1999). Integrated care: The impact of governmental behaviour on collaborative networks. *Health Policy, 49*, 149–159.

Mur-Veeman, I., van Raak, A., & Paulus, A. (2008). Comparing integrated care policy in Europe: Does policy matter? *Health Policy, 85*, 172–183. doi:10.1016/j.healthpol.2007.07.008

Murray, C. J. L., & Frenk, J. (2000). Theme papers: A framework for assessing the performance of health systems. *Bulletin of the World Health Organisation, 78(6)*, 728. doi:10.1590/S0042-96862000000600004

Najam, A. (2000). The four C's of government third sector-government relations. *Nonprofit Management and Leadership, 10*, 375–396. doi:10.1002/nml.10403

National Department of Health. (1997). *White Paper for the Transformation of the Health System in South Africa.* Pretoria: DoH.

National Department of Health. (2000). *The Primary Health Care Package for South Africa – A Set of Norms and Standards*. Pretoria: DoH.

National Department of Health. (2002). A District Hospital Service Package for South Africa: A Set of Norms and Standards. In. Pretoria: DoH.

National Department of Health. (2003). *Policy Guidelines on Child and Adolescent Mental Health*, Pretoria: NDoH.

National Department of Health. (2012a). *Policy Guideline on 72-hour Assessment of Involuntary Mental Health Care Users*. Pretoria: NDoH.

National Department of Health. (2012b). SA: Motsoaledi: Address by the Minister of Health, at the national mental health summit, Johannesburg (12/04/2012) [Press release]. Retrieved from www.polity.org.za/article/sa-motsoaledi-address-by-the-minister-of-heallth-at-the-national-mental-health-summit-johannesburg-12042012-2012-04-12 (accessed 7 May 2017).

National Department of Health. (2013). *National Mental Health Policy Framework and Strategic Plan 2013–2020*. Pretoria: NDoH.

National Mental Health Summit. (2012). The Ekurhuleni Declaration on Mental Health – April 2012. *African Journal of Psychiatry, 15*(6), 381–383.

Nattrass, N. (1996). Gambling on investment: Competing economic strategies in South Africa. *Transformation, 31*, 25–42.

Ndinda, C., Chilwane, D., & Mokomane, Z. (2013). *Civil society activism in accessing health care in South Africa: Technical report*. Developed for the Council for Social Science Development in Africa (CODESRIA), September 2013.

News24. (2020). 'Hands off our soup kitchens' – UN Women asked to stop SA govt interference in NPO work. *News24*. Retrieved from https://citizen.co.za/news/covid-19/2286057/hands-off-our-soup-kitchens-un-women-asked-to-stop-sa-govt-interference-in-npo-work/ (accessed 12 June 2020).

NGO Pulse. (2018). The three main lessons from Life Esidimeni according to Health Ombud. Retrieved from www.ngopulse.org/press-release/%E2%80%8B-three-main-lessons-life-esidimeni-according-health-ombud-0 (accessed 8 May 2019).

Ngo, V. K., Rubinstein, A., Ganju, V., Kanellis, P., Loza, N., Rabadan-Diehl, C., & Daar, A. S. (2013). Grand challenges: Integrating mental health care into the non-communicable disease agenda. *PLoS Medicine, 10*, 1–5. doi:10.1371/journal.pmed.1001443

Nicaise, P., Dubois, V., & Lorant, V. (2014). Mental health care delivery system reform in Belgium: The challenge of achieving deinstitutionalisation whilst addressing fragmentation of care at the same time. *Health Policy, 115*, 120–127. doi:10.1016/j.healthpol.2014.02.007

Nicaise, P., Tulloch, S., Dubois, V., Matanov, A., Priebe, S., & Lorant, V. (2013). Using social network analysis for assessing mental health and social services inter-organisational collaboration: Findings in deprived areas in Brussels and London. *Administration and Policy in Mental Health and Mental Health Services Research, 40*, 331–339. doi:10.1007/s10488-012-0423-y

Nilsen, E. R., Dugstad, J., Eide, H., Gullslett, M. K., & Eide, T. (2016). Exploring resistance to implementation of welfare technology in municipal health care services – a longitudinal case study. *BMC Health Services Research, 16*, 657. doi:10.1186/s12913-016-1913-5

Nosrati, E., & Marmot, M. (2019). Punitive social policy: An upstream determinant of health. *Lancet, 394*(10196), 376–377. doi:10.1016/s0140-6736(19)31672-1

Nussbaum, M. C. (1998). Victims and agents: What Greek tragedy can teach us about sympathy and responsibility. *Boston Review*, *23*, 21–24.

Organisation for Economic Cooperation and Development. (2008). *Paris Declaration on Aid Effectiveness and the Accra Agenda for Action*. Paris: OECD.

Ornellas, A., & Engelbrecht, L. K. (2018). The Life Esidimeni crisis: Why a neoliberal agenda leaves no room for the mentally ill. *Social Work*, *54*(3), 296–308.

Ouwens, M., Wollersheim, H. U. B., Hermens, R., & Hulscher, M. (2005). Integrated care programmes for chronically ill patients: A review of systematic reviews. *17*, 141–146.

Patel, V., Araya, R., Chatterjee, S., Chisholm, D., Cohen, A., De Silva, M., … van Ommeren, M. (2007). Treatment and prevention of mental disorders in low-income and middle-income countries. *Lancet, 370*, 991–1005. doi:10.1016/S0140-6736(07)61240–9

Patel, V., Belkin, G. S., Chockalingam, A., Cooper, J., Saxena, S., & Unützer, J. (2013). Grand challenges: Integrating mental health services into priority health care platforms. *PLoS Medicine, 10*. doi:10.1371/journal.pmed.1001448

Patel, V., Boyce, N., Collins, P. Y., Saxena, S., & Horton, R. (2011). A renewed agenda for global mental health. *The Lancet, 378*, 1441–1442. doi:10.1016/S0140-6736(11)61385-8

Patel, V. et al. (2015). Global priorities for addressing the burden of mental, neurological, and substance use disorders. In V. Patel et al. (Eds.), *Mental, Neurological, and Substance Use Disorders: Disease Control Priorities* (3rd ed., pp. 1–27). Washington, DC: World Bank Group.

Patel, V., & Saxena, S. (2014). Transforming lives, enhancing communities – innovations in global mental health. *New England Journal of Medicine, 370*, 498–501. doi:10.1056/NEJMp1313771

Patton, P. (2014). Foucault and Rawls: Government and public reason. In V. Lemm & M. Vatter (Eds.), *The Government of Life Foucault, Biopolitics, and Neoliberalism* (pp. 141–162). New York: Fordham University Press.

Paulson, G. (2012). *Closing the Asylums: Causes and Consequences of the Deinstitutionalization Movement*. Jefferson, MD: McFarland.

Peet, R. (2002). Ideology, discourse, and the geography of hegemony: From socialist to neoliberal development in postapartheid South Africa. *Antipode, 34*, 54–84.

Petersen, I. (2000). Comprehensive integrated primary mental health care for South Africa. Pipedream or possibility? *Social Science & Medicine, 51*, 321–334. doi:http://dx.doi.org/10.1016/S0277-9536(99)00456-6

Petersen, I., & Lund, C. (2011). Mental health service delivery in South Africa from 2000 to 2010: One step forward, one step back. *South African Medical Journal, 101*(10), 751–757.

Petersen, I., Lund, C., Bhana, A., & Flisher, A. J. (2012). A task shifting approach to primary mental health care for adults in South Africa: Human resource requirements and costs for rural settings. *Health Policy and Planning, 27*, 42–51. doi:10.1093/heapol/czr012

Petersen, I., Lund, C., & Stein, D. J. (2011). Optimizing mental health services in low-income and middle-income countries. *Current Opinion in Psychiatry, 24*, 318–323. doi:10.1097/YCO.0b013e3283477afb

Petersen, I., Marais, D., Abdulmalik, J., Ahuja, S., Alem, A., Chisholm, D., … Thornicroft, G. (2017a). Strengthening mental health system governance in six low- and middle-income countries in Africa and South Asia: Challenges, needs and potential strategies. doi:10.1093/heapol/czx014

Petersen, I., Marais, D., Abdulmalik, J., Ahuja, S., Alem, A., Chisholm, D., … Thornicroft, G. (CC). Strengthening mental health system governance in six low- and middle-income countries in Africa and South Asia: Challenges, needs and potential strategies. *Health Policy and Planning, 32*, 699–709. doi:10.1093/heapol/czx014

Petersen, I., van Rensburg, A., Gigaba, S., Luvuno, Z. P. B., & Fairall, L. (2020). Health systems strengthening to optimise scale-up in global mental health in low- and middle-income countries: Lessons from the frontlines. *Epidemiol Psychiatr Sci, 29*, e101. doi:10.1017/s2045796020000141

Pickersgill, M. D. (2012). What is psychiatry? Co-producing complexity in mental health. *Social Theory & Health, 10*(4): 328–347. doi:10.1057/sth.2012.9.

Pickersgill, M. D. (2013). Debating DSM-5: diagnosis and the sociology of critique. *Journal of Medical Ethics, 40*(8): 521–525. doi:10.1136/medethics-2013-101762.

Piketty, T. (2014). *Capital in the Twenty-First Century*. Cambridge, MA: Harvard University Press.

Plagerson, S. (2015). Integrating mental health and social development in theory and practice. *Health Policy and Planning, 30*, 163–170. doi:10.1093/heapol/czt107

Polanyi, K. (1977). The economistic fallacy. *Review (Fernand Braudel Center), 1*(1), 9–18.

Postle, K., & Beresford, P. (2007). Capacity building and the reconception of political participation: A role for social care workers? *British Journal of Social Work, 37*, 143–158.

Power, M. (2000). The audit society – second thoughts. *International Journal of Auditing, 4*, 111–119. doi:10.1111/1099–1123.00306

Poyner, J. (2009). *JM Coetzee and the Paradox of Postcolonial Authorship*. Farnham: Ashgate Publishing Limited.

Provan, K. G., Ark, M., Veazie, A., Staten, L. K., Icolette, N., & Teufel-Shone, I. (2005). The use of network analysis to strengthen community partnerships. *Public Administration Review, 65*, 603–613.

Purdy, J. M. (2012). A framework for assessing power in collaborative governance processes. *Public Administration Review, 72*, 409–417. doi:10.1111/j.1540-6210.2011.02525.x

QSR International (2016). NVivo qualitative data analysis software. QSR International Pty Ltd. Version 10.

Raffnsøe, S., Gudmand-Høyer, M., & Thaning, M. S. (2016). *Michel Foucault: A Research Companion*. Basingstoke: Palgrave Macmillan.

Ramlall, S., Chipps, J., & Mars, M. (2010). Impact of the South African Mental Health Care Act No. 17 of 2002 on regional and district hospitals designated for mental health care in KwaZulu-Natal. *South African Medical Journal, 100*(10), 667–670.

Rathod, S., Pinninti, N., Irfan, M., Gorczynski, P., Gega, L., Rathod, P., & Naeem, F. (2017). Mental health service provision in low- and middle-income countries. *Health Services Insights, 10*. doi:10.1177/1178632917694350

Rawls, J. (1971). *A Theory of Justice*. Cambridge, MA: Harvard University Press.

Rawls, J. (1999). *The Law of Peoples: The Idea of Public Reason Revisited*. Cambridge, MA: Harvard University Press.

Rawls, J. (2001). *Justice as Fairness: A Restatement*. Cambridge, MA: Harvard University Press.

Rispel, L. & Setswei, G. (2007). Stewardship: Protecting the public's health. In S. Harrison, R. Bhana, & A. Ntuli, (Eds.), *South African Health Review* (pp. 3–17). Durban: Human Services Research Council.

Robertson, L. J., & Szabo, C. P. (2017). Community mental health services in Southern Gauteng: An audit using Gauteng District Health Information Systems data. *2017, 23*. doi:10.4102/sajpsychiatry.v23i0.1055

Rochefort, D. (1997). *From Poorhouses to Homelessness: Policy Analysis and Mental Health care*. Dover, MA: Auburn House.

Rose, N. (1996a) Governing "advanced" liberal democracies. In A. Barry, T. Osborne, and N. Rose, (Eds.), *Foucault and Political Reason: Liberalism, Neo-liberalism and Rationalities of Government* (pp. 37–64). Chicago: University of Chicago Press.

Rose, N. (1996b). Psychiatry as a political science: Advanced liberalism and the administration of risk. *History of the Human Sciences, 9*, 1–23. doi:10.1177/095269519600900201

Rose, N. (1999). Powers of rreedom: Re-framing political thought. doi:http://dx.doi.org/10.1017/CB09780511488856

Rose, N. (2003). Neurochemical selves. *Society, 41*(1), 46–59. doi:10.1007/bf02688204

Rose, N. (2019). *Our Psychiatric Future: The Politics of Mental Health*. Cambridge: Polity Press.

Rose, N., & Miller, P. (2010a). Political power beyond the state: Problematics of government. *British Journal of Sociology, 61*, 271–303. doi:10.1111/j.1468-4446.2009.01247.x

Rosenberg, A., Hartwig, K., & Merson, M. (2008). Government-NGO collaboration and sustainability of orphans and vulnerable children projects in southern Africa. *Evaluation and Program Planning, 31*(1), 51–60. doi:10.1016/j.evalprogplan.2007.08.005

Rotarou, E. S., & Sakellariou, D. (2017). Inequalities in access to health care for people with disabilities in Chile: The limits of universal health coverage. *Critical Public Health, 27*(5), 604–616. doi:10.1080/09581596.2016.1275524

Roy, A. (2020, 3 April 2020). Arundhati Roy: "The pandemic is a portal". *Financial Times*. Retrieved from www.ft.com/content/10d8f5e8-74eb-11ea-95fe-fcd274e920ca (accessed 5 April 2020).
Rummery, K. (2009). Healthy partnerships, healthy citizens? An international review of partnerships in health and social care and patient/user outcomes. *Social Science and Medicine, 69*, 1797–1804. doi:10.1016/j.socscimed.2009.09.004
Saldaña, J. (2014). Coding and analysis strategies. In P. Leavy, (Ed.), *The Oxford Handbook of Qualitative Research* (pp. 581–605). Oxford: Oxford University Press.
Saltman, R. B., & Ferroussier-Davis, O. (2000). The concept of stewardship in health policy. *Bulletin of the World Health Organization, 78*, 732–739. doi:10.1590/S0042-96862000000600005
Santermans, L., Zeeuws, D., Vanderbruggen, N., & Crunelle, C. L. (2019). Mobile crisis team in the brussels region: Facts and figures. *Psychiatria Danubina, 31*(Suppl 3), 418–420.
Saraceno, B., & Dua, T. (2009). Global mental health: The role of psychiatry. *European Archives of Psychiatry and Clinical Neuroscience, 259*, S109–S117.
Satgar, V. (2012). Beyond Marikana: The post-apartheid South African State. *Africa Spectrum, 47*(2–3), 33–62. doi:10.1177/000203971204702-303
Savage, G. T., Taylor, R. L., Rotarius, T. M., & Buesseler, J. A. (1997). Governance of integrated delivery systems/networks: A stakeholder approach. *Health Care Management Review, 22*, 7–20. doi:10.1097/00004010-199701000-00002
Scott, B. (2016). *The Cultural Hegemony of Mental Health*, Bella Caledonia, 22 September. Retrieved from https://bellacaledonia.org.uk/2016/09/22/the-cultural-hegemony-of-mental-health/ (accessed 3 May 2017).
Scott, V., Schaay, N., Olckers, P., Nqana, N., Lehmann, U., & Gilson, L. (2014). Exploring the nature of governance at the level of implementation for health system strengthening: The DIALHS experience. *Health Policy and Planning, 29*, ii59–ii70. doi:10.1093/heapol/czu073
Seekings, J. (2020, 2 June). Feeding poor people: The national government has failed. *GroundUp*. Retrieved from www.groundup.org.za/article/feeding-poor-people-national-government-has-failed/ (accessed 5 June 2020).
Semrau, M., Evans-Lacko, S., Alem, A., Ayuso-Mateos, J. L., Chisholm, D., Gureje, O., … Thornicroft, G. (2015). Strengthening mental health systems in low- and middle-income countries: The Emerald programme. 1–9. doi:10.1186/s12916-015-0309-4
Sennett, R. (2003). *Respect: The Formation of Character in an Age of Inequality*. London: Penguin Books.
Sennett, R. (2006). *The Culture of the New Capitalism*. New Haven: Yale University Press.
Shen, G. C., & Snowden, L. R. (2014). Institutionalization of deinstitutionalization: A cross-national analysis of mental health system reform. *International Journal of Mental Health Systems, 8*, 47. doi:10.1186/1752-4458-8-47
Sheth, H. (2009). Deinstitutionalization or disowning responsibility. *International Journal of Psychosocial Rehabilitation, 13*, 11–20.
Simon, J. (2011). *From the Medical Model to the Humanitarian Crisis Model: California's Prison Health Crisis and the Future of Imprisonment*. Paper presented at the Reflecting on 20 years of The Foucault Effect: Studies in Governmentality, Birkbeck College, University of London. https://backdoorbroadcasting.net/2011/06/jonathan-simon-from-the-medical-model-to-the-humanitarian-crisis-model-californias-prison-health-crisis-and-the-future-of-imprisonment/ (accessed 12 December 2019).

Sitas, A. (2010). *The Mandela Decade 1990–2000: Labour, Culture and Society in Post-Apartheid South Africa.* Pretoria: UNISA Press.

Sontag, S. (1978). *Illness as metaphor*. New York: Farrar, Straus and Giroux.

Sontag, S. (1989). *AIDS and its metaphors*. New York: Farrar, Straus and Giroux.

Sorsdahl, K., Stein, D. J., Grimsrud, A., Seedat, S., Flisher, A. J., Williams, D. R., & Myer, L. (2009). Traditional healers in the treatment of common mental disorders in South Africa. *The Journal of Nervous and Mental Disease, 197*, 434–441. doi:10.1097/NMD.0b013e3181a61dbc

South African Government (1996). *Constitution of the Republic of South Africa.* Pretoria: Government Printer.

South African Government (1997a). *Non-Profit Organisations Act.* Pretoria: Government Printer.

South African Government (1997b). *Non-Profit Organisations Act, 1997*. Pretoria: Government Printer

South African Government (2002). *Mental Health Care Act No 17 of 2002*. Pretoria: Government Printer.

South African Government (2004). *The National Health Act No 61 of 2003*. Pretoria: Government Printer.

South African Government. (2015). *Marikana Commission of Inquiry: Report on Matters of Public, National and International Concern Arising out of the Tragic Incidents at the Lonmin Mine in Marikana, in the North West Province*. Pretoria: Government Gazette No. 699 of 2015, 81/172488 (Z 19E).

South African Human Rights Commission. (2017). *Report of the National Hearing on the Status of Mental Health Care in South Africa*. Pretoria: SAHRC.

Springer, S. (2012). Neoliberalism as discourse: Between Foucauldian political economy and Marxian poststructuralism. *Critical Discourse Studies, 9*(2), 133–147. doi:10.1080/17405904.2012.656375

Stanley, E. (2001). Evaluating the truth and reconciliation commission. *The Journal of Modern African Studies, 39*(3), 525–546.

Statistics South Africa (2009). *Financial Statistics of National Government 2007/2008*. Pretoria: StatsSA.

Statistics South Africa (2016). *Community Survey 2016: Provinces at a Glance*. Pretoria: StatsSA.

Statistics South Africa. (2019). *Financial Statistics of National Government 2017/2018*. Pretoria: StatsSA.

Stein, D. J. (2014). A new mental health policy for South Africa. *SAMJ: South African Medical Journal, 104*(2), 115–116.

Stein, D. J., Williams, D. R., & Kessler, R. C. (2009). The South African Stress and Health (SASH) study: A scientific base for mental health policy. *SAMJ: South African Medical Journal, 99*(5), 337–337.

Sturmberg, J. P., & Njoroge, A. (2017). People-centred health systems, a bottom-up approach: Where theory meets empery. *Journal of Evaluation in Clinical Practice, 23*(2), 467–473.

Swartz, S. (1995). The black insane in the Cape, 1891–1920. *Journal of Southern African Studies, 21*(3), 399–415.

Swartz, S. (1995). Colonizing the insane: Causes of insanity in the Cape, 1891–1920. *History of the Human Sciences, 8*(4), 39–57.

Swartz, S. (2009). Madness and method: Approaches to the history of mental illness. *Psychology in Society, 37*: 70–74.

Sylvestre, J., Nelson, G., & Aubry, T. (2017). *Advances in community psychology: Housing, citizenship, and communities for people with serious mental illness: Theory, research, practice, and policy perspectives*. Oxford: Oxford University Press.

Szabo, C. P., & Kaliski, S. Z. (2017). Mental health and the law: A South African perspective. *BJPsych international, 14*(3), 69–71.

Teghtsoonian, K. (2009). Depression and mental health in neoliberal times: A critical analysis of policy and discourse. *Social Science & Medicine, 69*(1), 28–35. doi:https://doi.org/10.1016/j.socscimed.2009.03.037

Terreblanche, S. (1999) *The Ideological Journey of South Africa: From the RDP to the GEAR Macro-economic Plan*. Cape Town: University of Cape Town.

Thornicroft, G., Deb, T., & Henderson, C. (2016). Community mental health care worldwide: current status and further developments. *World psychiatry: official journal of the World Psychiatric Association (WPA), 15*, 276–286. doi:10.1002/wps.20349

Thornicroft, G., & Patel, V. (2014). Including mental health among the new sustainable development goals. *BMJ, 349*, g5189-g5189. doi:10.1136/bmj.g5189

Thornicroft, G., & Tansella, M. (2002). Balancing community-based and hospital-based mental health care. *World Psychiatry, 1*, 84–90.

Tomlinson, M., & Lund, C. (2012). Why does mental health not get the attention it deserves? An application of the Shiffman and Smith framework. *PLoS Medicine, 9*(2), e1001178-e1001178. doi:10.1371/journal.pmed.1001178

Tomlinson, M., Rudan, I., Saxena, S., Swartz, L., Tsaid, A. C., & Patel, V. (2009). Setting priorities for global mental health research. *Bulletin of the World Health Organization, 87*, 438–446. doi:10.2471/BLT.08.054353

Torkelson, E. (2017). There's a problem with the CPS grant payment system that Minister Bathabile Dlamini isn't talking about. *Huffington Post*, 7 March.

Ure, G. B. (2015). *A hermeneutical analysis of the impact of socio-political and legislative developments on South African institutional mental health care from 1904 to 2004*. PhD diss., University of the Witwatersrand, Johannesburg.

Vahia, V. N. (2013). Diagnostic and statistical manual of mental disorders 5: A quick glance. *Indian Journal of Psychiatry, 55*(3), 220–223. doi:10.4103/0019-5545.117131

Valentijn, P. P., Boesveld, I. C., Van der Klauw, D. M., Ruwaard, D., Struijs, J. N., Molema, J. J. W., … Vrijhoef, H. J. (2015). Towards a taxonomy for integrated care: A mixed-methods study. *International Journal of Integrated Care, 15*, 1–18. doi:10.5334/ijic.1513

Valentijn, P. P., Schepman, S. M., Opheij, W., & Bruijnzeels, M. A. (2013). Understanding integrated care: A comprehensive conceptual framework based on the integrative functions of primary care. *International Journal of Integrated Care, 13*. doi:10.5334/ijic.886

Van den Heever, A. (2011). *Evaluation of the Green Paper on National Health Insurance*. Submission to the National Department of Health.

Van den Heever, A. (2012). *Review of Competition in the South African Health System*. Johannesburg: Produced for the Competition Commission.

van der Westhuizen, C., Myers, B., Malan, M., Naledi, T., Roelofse, M., Stein, D. J., … Sorsdahl, K. (2019). Implementation of a screening, brief intervention and referral to treatment programme for risky substance use in South African emergency centres: A mixed methods evaluation study. *PLOS ONE, 14*(11), e0224951. doi:10.1371/journal.pone.0224951 van Hulzen, K. J., Scholz, C. J., Franke, B., Ripke, S., Klein, M., McQuillin, A., … Andreassen, O. A. (2017). Genetic overlap between attention-deficit/hyperactivity disorder and bipolar disorder: evidence from genome-wide association study meta-analysis. *Biological psychiatry, 82*(9), 634–641.

Van Pletzen, E., Zulliger, R., Moshabela, M., & Schneider, H. (2013). The size, characteristics and partnership networks of the health-related non-profit sector in three regions of South Africa: Implications of changing primary health care policy for community-based care. *Health Policy and Planning, 29*, 742–752. doi:10.1093/heapol/czt058

van Pletzen, E., Zulliger, R., Moshabela, M., & Schneider, H. (2014). The size, characteristics and partnership networks of the health-related non-profit sector in three regions of South Africa: Implications of changing primary health care policy for community-based care. *Health Policy Plan, 29*(6), 742–752. doi:10.1093/heapol/czt058

van Rensburg, A. J., & Fourie, P. (2016). Health policy and integrated mental health care in the SADC region: Strategic clarification using the Rainbow Model. *International Journal of Mental Health Systems, 10*. doi:10.1186/s13033-016-0081-7

Van Rensburg, H. (2012). National health care systems: Structure, dynamics and types. In H. Van Rensburg (Ed.), *Health and Health Care in South Africa* (2nd ed., pp. 1–60). Pretoria: Van Schaik Publishers.

Van Rensburg, H., & Engelbrecht, M. (2012a). Transformation of the South African health system: Post-1994. In H. Van Rensburg (Ed.), *Health and Health Care in South Africa* (2nd ed.). Pretoria: Van Schaik Publishers.

Van Zyl Slabbert, F. (2006). *The Other Side of History: An Anecdotal Reflection on Political Transition in South Africa*. Johannesburg: Jonathan Ball Publishers.

Visser, W. (2005). Shifting RDP into gear: The ANC government's dilemma in providing an equitable system of social security for the "new" South Africa. *ITH-Tagungsberichte 39 "Mercy or Right". Development of Social Security Systems, Akademische Verlaganstalt, Wien*, 105–124.

Wacquant, L. (2008). The place of the prison in the New Government of Poverty. In M. L. Frampton, I. J. Lopez, & J. Simon (Eds.), *After the War on Crime: Race, Democracy, and a New Reconstruction* (pp. 23–36). New York: New York University Press.

Wacquant, L. (2009a). *Bringing the Penal State Back In*. London: London School of Economics.

Wacquant, L. (2009b). *Punishing the Poor: The Neoliberal Government of Social Insecurity*. Durham, NC: Duke University Press.

Wacquant, L. (2010). Crafting the neoliberal state: Workfare, prisonfare, and social insecurity. *Sociological Forum, 25*, 197–220. doi:10.1111/j.1573-7861.2010.01173.x

Wainberg, M. L., Scorza, P., Shultz, J. M., Helpman, L., Mootz, J. J., Johnson, K. A., … Arbuckle, M. R. (2017). Challenges and opportunities in global mental health: A research-to-practice perspective. *Current Psychiatry Reports, 19*, 28. doi:10.1007/s11920-017-0780-z

Wanna, J. (2008) Collaborative government: Meanings, dimensions, drivers and outcomes. In J. O'Flynn, & J. Wanna (Eds.), *Collaborative Governance: A New Era of Public Policy in Australia?* (pp. 3–22). Canberra: The Australian National University E Press.

Weber, M. (1947). *From Max Weber: Essays in Sociology*. New York: Oxford University Press.

Weinstein, H. M., & Stover, E. (2004). Introduction: Conflict, justice and reclamation. In E. Stover & H. M. Weinstein (Eds.), *My Neighbor, My Enemy: Justice and Community in the Aftermath of Mass Atrocity* (pp. 1–26). Cambridge: Cambridge University Press.

West, R. (1979, 9 June). Mulder and the mental hospitals. *The Spectator.*

Wihlman, U., Lundborg, C. S., Axelsson, R., & Holmström, I. (2008). Barriers of inter-organisational integration in vocational rehabilitation. *International Journal of Integrated Care, 8*, e52.

Willem, A., & Lucidarme, S. (2014). Pitfalls and challenges for trust and effectiveness in collaborative networks. *Public Management Review, 16*, 733–760. doi:10.1080/14719037.2012.744426

Wölfer, R., Faber, N. S., & Hewstone, M. (2015). Social network analysis in the science of groups: Cross-sectional and longitudinal applications for studying intra- and intergroup behavior. *Group Dynamics: Theory, Research, and Practice, 19*, 45–61.

Wolvaardt, G., van Niftrik, J., Beira, B., Mapham, W., & Tienie, S. (2008). The role of private and other non-governmental organisations in primary health care. *South African Health Review,* 223–236.

Woolford, A., & Curran, A. (2012). Community positions, neoliberal dispositions: Managing nonprofit social services within the bureaucratic field. *Critical Sociology, 39*, 45–63.

World Bank (2020). Civil society. Retrieved from www.worldbank.org/en/about/partners/civil-society/overview (accessed 24 June 2020).

World Health Organization (2000). *The World Health Report 2000: Health Systems: Improving Performance*. Geneva: WHO.

World Health Organization (2008). *Integrating Mental Health into Primary Care: A Global Perspective*. Geneva: WHO.

World Health Organization, African National Congress, & United Nations Children's Fund (1994). *A National Health Plan for South Africa*. Johannesburg: African National Congress.

Yin, R. K. (2009). *Case Study Research: Design and Methods.* Thousand Oaks, CA: Sage.

Žižek, S. (2010). A permanent economic emergency. *New Left Review, 64*, 85–95.

Index

Note: Page numbers in *italics* indicate figures and in **bold** indicate tables on the corresponding pages.

For Product Safety Concerns and Information please contact our EU
representative GPSR@taylorandfrancis.com
Taylor & Francis Verlag GmbH, Kaufingerstraße 24, 80331 München, Germany

www.ingramcontent.com/pod-product-compliance
Lightning Source LLC
Chambersburg PA
CBHW060308220326
41598CB00027B/4272
* 9 7 8 0 3 6 7 6 8 3 2 9 0 *